Diabetes Winning Strategies and Keto Cookbook

Who Says You Can't Lower Blood Sugar to Normal and Live Healthier – 70 Delicious Keto Recipes Inside!

(2 Manuscripts)

DAVID F. WILSON
ANIVYA PUBLISHING

CONTENTS

MANUSCRIPT - 2: The Keto Cookbook

DIABETES WINNING STRATEGIES AND KETO COOKBOOK

There are no guarantees of income to be made, traffic delivered or other promises of any kind. Readers are cautioned to rely on their own judgment about their individual circumstances and to act accordingly. By reading any document, the reader agrees that under no circumstances is the author responsible for any losses, direct or indirect, that are incurred as a result of use of the information contained within this document, including - but not limited to errors, omissions, or inaccuracies.

INTRODUCTION

Diabetes. The disease is prolific and more people are contracting it. According to the ***American Diabetes Association***, here are some alarming statistics:

- Almost 30 million children and adults in the United States have diabetes.

- 86 million Americans have pre-diabetes.

- 1.4 million Americans are diagnosed with diabetes every year.

- People die on average at least 6 years sooner than those without the disease.

Does this mean that diabetes is growing out of control? Why is this happening? Here's what ***Harvard Health*** had to say:

"Diabetes has been on the upswing since the 1960s, fueled largely by Americans' penchant for eating too much and exercising too little. The combination of excess weight and inactivity makes tissues resistant to insulin, which snowballs into diabetes. **The CDC's new warning factors in** the continuing spread of obesity and inactivity with the aging of the U.S. population, the higher risk for diabetes in rapidly growing minority populations, and improvements in medical care that help people with diabetes live longer."

If these alarming facts are of concern to you, just imagine what the world will look like in another 20 years. Diabetes is currently affecting over 371 million people worldwide. If projections hold we could see double the number of people develop diabetes in just the next twenty years alone . . . Yet there is hope for sufferers.

That is what this eBook is all about: hope, change and modern research. There are ways to improve your life as a diabetic, **to finally limit or even fully suppress diabetes** so as to lessen its impact and destructive force.

Let's take this journey together right now.

WHAT REALLY IS DIABETES?

Diabetes is an often-misunderstood "disease" and is NOT what you may have been told it is. Here is the typical generic description of what diabetes is said to be, to start our discussion:

di·a·be·tes

/ˌdīəˈbēdēz, ˌdīəˈbēdis/

noun

a metabolic disease in which the body's inability to produce any or enough insulin causes elevated levels of glucose in the blood.

As you can see, this is a standard definition, simply explained and it even makes sense. Yet it is NOT what diabetes *really* is. . .

If there was a proper definition, one that had a solution or potential treatment for the disease, science would have described it this way: **"Diabetes is a form of intoxication (poison) that is the result of toxic overload of your cells which interferes with your body's ability to produce insulin."** – My quote and it is the BEST definition.

Diabetes is like being poisoned? YES. The term intoxication actually is used to describe poisoning, such as the term *foodborne intoxication*. So, let's take a look at the definition of foodborne intoxication (yes, this will all make sense soon):

"Foodborne infection is caused by the ingestion of food containing live bacteria which grow and establish themselves in the human intestinal tract. **Foodborne intoxication is caused by ingesting food containing toxins** formed by bacteria which resulted from the bacterial growth in the food item."

Source: http://food.unl.edu/food-poisoning-foodborne-illness

What do you notice here? A foodborne illness *results in an intoxication* that affects the entire body, makes you sick and will continue making you sick until the bacteria / toxins leave your body.

I am here to say that **Diabetes is CAUSED by toxins** in your food. Some of those toxins are sugar, but mostly they are contaminants in food, water, air and the myriad of chemicals we are all exposed to daily. These toxins bio – accumulate (which is why we become pre-diabetic first) until your body can no longer regulate blood glucose.

When you eat enough toxic food, your body begins to break down.

When toxins build up in your body, things begin to go wrong. This will destroy the body's ability to self-regulate, especially at a cellular level.

This is because toxins **burn out control receptors in**

your cells and over time cause a gradual reduction in the ability to control many hormones in the body, including insulin production and insulin resistance. Modern medicine says there is no cure for diabetes and while that is technically true (medicine does not recognize holistic medicine), there are ways to suppress the disease so much, it has no impact on your life.

WHY THERE IS NO MEDICAL CURE – FOLLOW THE MONEY

Recently I read an article saying scientists are claiming type I diabetes (essentially insulin dependent) is now quite possibly reversible in time:

". . .type 1 diabetes has long been thought to be a permanent condition that requires lifelong insulin dependence. Excitingly, a new study published just last month suggests that a 'fasting mimicking diet" could effectively reverse the pathology of type 1 diabetes in mice."

Over the years I have seen hundreds of related studies and information by researchers that indicate the scientific community not only KNOWS diabetes is reversible, but that there are also many "folk cures" that have been completely discounted by our society.

Why is this the case for diabetics? Most people

already know the answer:

"If you are a diabetes patient, you are Big Pharma's best friend. **You have been earmarked for the rest of your life as a cash cow** for the companies who make diabetes medicines, syringes, blood sugar monitors, insulin, cotton swabs, and more. But there is a little secret that the pharmaceutical companies don't want you to know."

The 'secret' is that YOU are capable of eliminating pre-diabetes and type II diabetes all on your own. You can suppress type I diabetes and, in some cases, 'cure' the disease (almost complete suppression) just with over the counter products that are cheap, and that I will share with you -- as well as multiple folk 'cures' that have been used for over a hundred years and seem to work better than pharmaceutical drugs.

According to today's researchers, cures for diabetes have **been hidden from the general public for over 40 years** because as soon as a cure is developed, companies that produce diabetic drugs and supplies will purchase this research / information to keep it quiet:

"There are numerous examples of well-educated, innovative doctors and scientists who have created alternative medical treatments that far supersede conventional drug treatments, and yet they are more frequently than not shunned, persecuted, or even prosecuted for their efforts." - Dr. Mercola

Follow the money could not be truer here.

So now you know that big corporations drive commerce by banking on disease maintenance but NOT curatives.

Think about it: why should any corporation making literally BILLIONS of dollars a year (471 BILLION on average yearly in this market) ever want to find a cure? Drug companies *make customers not cures* and if you are one of the customers, I strongly suggest you take your health strongly in your own hands.

PEOPLE ARE WAKING UP TO THIS ONGOING SCAM.

Now the drug companies see that there is blood in the water over this issue so they are finally being compelled to release a cure; even if that 'cure' creates more health issues and with big Pharma, you can bet it will.

A DIABETIC'S DEFINITION OF DIABETES

Remember what I said about the definition of Diabetes? Diabetes is a form of **toxic overload** that affects your pancreas, liver, gallbladder, and kidneys. The organs become so toxic that over time, they malfunction and eventually replicate malfunctioning cells. As these cells propagate (much like cancer) your body begins a slow decline until Diabetes appears.

The lack of properly functioning cells **is at the heart of many diseases** (i.e. Cancer) and if you are diabetic, you have increased likelihood of developing other secondary illnesses and conditions too.

Nice, huh? Believe me I hated this as well. I was so MAD when I discovered that I have been lied to by:

- **My parents** (who did not know diabetes can be reversed).

- **My friends** (who did not know diabetes can be reversed).

- **My College** (who did not know diabetes can be reversed).

- **My health care provider HMO** (diabetes is not reversible according to them)

- **My doctor** (doctors no longer receive training in holistic medicine, just how to prescribe drugs).

- **The hospital** (who did not know diabetes can be reversed)..

Are we seeing a trend here? If you look long enough you will find the fingerprints of big Pharma all over the diabetes lies. Now is the time to take back your health and do so in a way that thousands of sufferers have discovered.

Is Your Food Toxic? Yes . .

Now we can clearly see that all the hype that is directed at diabetics, especially from the medical industry, is not only unwarranted **but does not take into consideration the highly toxic diet that is being foisted on us** by large corporations who care nothing about our health and only want to sell all of their crappy junk foods.

As a former diabetic, I've been lectured by:

- ✓ Dietitians insisting I remain on a low-fat diet with few carbs. This is despite the fact that low-fat diets are now being proven to cause illness and that we NEED more high quality fats to survive.

- ✓ My doctor who insisted the solution is more diabetic drugs and maintenance as opposed to any attempt at a "cure."

- ✓ Most people in general telling me I need to follow their advice on diet and exercise and stop being lazy, even though a majority of them are pre-diabetic or toxic or both too . .
    .

So now we know that despite all the lies we hear about diabetes, that the biggest problem we have is a society *filled with toxins* in our food, air, water, medicine, cosmetics etc.

It is quite possible to be exposed to **thousands of chemicals DAILY** that are laced throughout every aspect of our society that we are exposed to!

These chemicals will make you sick over time and unfortunately most of us are not aware that we are consuming them every day in one form or another. Currently you must devise a way to avoid *at least* 80% of the toxic foods, chemicals and additives that you are exposed to on a regular basis. This is the only way to reverse the damage that has been done, which will bring us into our next section in the guide.

STOP EATING JUNK FOODS!

Even if you're not aware of it, *diabetes and the complications* that you experience are now factored to be the seventh leading cause of death in the United States and number 6 worldwide:

What is interesting to note from the chart above is that **every form of death that is experienced**, with the exception of road injury, can be directly or indirectly linked to a junk diet filled with toxin-laden foods!

Diabetes is the seventh leading killer in the United States and number six worldwide, -- you now know this. Those statistics alone are reason enough to invest time and research into also seeing that the majority of related diseases are also part of our studies.

More research is emerging daily that suggests that almost all forms of illness that we experience in a modern society are directly linked to a junk food diet, lack of exercise, lack of proper nutrients and the pressure cooker, super stressful society we all live in.

Can there be any reason *not to see that we are all being poisoned* and many of us are willing participants in our own illnesses? For example, just one "sweetener," aspartame could be one of the worst poisons ever concocted by man, yet it is everywhere in our food chain:

"Aspartame is a neurotoxin. Even ants have sense enough to avoid it. Yet, diet drinks and many foods add this neurotoxin chemical as its sweetener, and they promote it as a heath food to a public that naively puts its trust in the experts. Drink water. Drink tea. Drink regular soda – anything but the diet sodas. You just might live longer." –Dr. Mercola

It's not just toxins like aspartame in your food that we have to watch out for **but all forms of toxins** that are used to process foods:

 "A report by the Union of Concerned Scientists estimates that 70 percent of antibiotics used in this country are given to animals for growth promotion and other non-medical uses. And when all agricultural uses were considered, they estimated the share could be as high as 84 percent! This massive antibiotic overuse is largely responsible for the potent strains of antibiotic-resistant bacteria we are seeing today." –Dr. Mercola

Perhaps the only way to achieve a completely healthy lifestyle is to make sure all food that passes your lips is wholesome, 100% truly organic and in a form that has not been processed in any way.

Even if you manage to get this type of food, the word 'organic' has changed over the years to just mean most foods grown in the ground. It is also supposed to mean that pesticides and other toxins are not used, but that is not always the case:

HOW ONE MAN REVERSED HIS DIABETES – HIS DOCTOR WAS STUNNED!

I wanted to first give you enough background information on diabetes and the connection to **poor food choices,** and the toxins that they contain, as the main reason why you might be suffering with diabetes.

In addition, you may want to ask me why the heck you should listen to what I have to say. Well that is a good question.

I want to explain to you that I fully understand what you're going through because I have experienced it for many years:

- ✓ Often uncontrolled blood glucose readings as high as 400.

- ✓ Diabetic secondary conditions like nerve pain.

- ✓ Heavy thirst and a need to void often (pee).

- ✓ Slow healing ulcers (wounds on the skin) and related pain.

I understand all the things that you're going through, but I want to tell you my story because **it involves a new mindset** in a way that you can take charge of your disease and eventually reverse most, if not all, of the damage and finally gain control over diabetes.

I started out many years ago like most people.

Even though I only ate twice a day I was overweight, unhappy and unhealthy. For many years and couldn't understand why it was difficult to lose weight and I began to notice some diabetic complications.

After visiting my doctor, I was told that I was having issues controlling my blood sugar and that there is a good chance that I was a diabetic and might require insulin.

At the time I knew very little about diabetes and believed all the lies I was told. I was told that I contracted the disease primarily because I consumed large quantities of sugar.

I knew this was untrue.

Yet it wasn't the sugar that I was eating too much of. I had a love of diet Pepsi, which I believe was the reason why I contracted diabetes:

"Research by the Karolinska Institute on 2,800 adults found that those who consumed at least two

200ml servings of soft drinks daily were 2.4 times as likely to suffer from a form of type 2 diabetes."

Other studies have confirmed that diet soft drinks contain aspartame and/or other types of artificial sweeteners that damage your cells' ability to regulate glucose levels; and new studies show it makes you FAT.

As mentioned earlier, as toxins bio-accumulate in the body, the body begins to break down and cells no longer recognize hormones that control sugar. As more cells become corrupted, the process continues progressively until diseases begin to appear.

It took me about three years of using diabetic medications to come to the realization that my body was not getting better and that the health decreases continued to spiral out of control.

It was at this point that I decided I needed to consider a holistic approach because I had heard of people curing their own diabetes.

IT ISN'T A "CURE" BUT IT IS VERY CLOSE

When I began my initial research into some type of **"folk cure,"** I started by researching diabetes websites, discussion groups, and reading magazines, medical journals, and white papers. I also studied "holistic curatives." Just about anything that was peer reviewed, I would read.

I was particularly interested in what average everyday people were doing to control, suppress or otherwise greatly reduce the effects of diabetes in their life.

I noticed that no doctor that writes prescriptions on a regular basis will agree that diabetes can be "cured" even though research is emerging to the contrary.

Once we understand what the premise of diabetes is, we can begin to see an actual methodology that will suppress the disease with very little work and no impact on your daily life.

Even though doctors will not readily admit that the disease can be 100% cured, **there can be little question that almost any disease under the right conditions in the human body can at least be suppressed** to a point that it can be completely controlled.

Few doctors will argue this point as disease suppression is a wonderful new field of study and it is gaining steam with all diseases.

Your immune system essentially does the same thing every single day; it suppresses disease to a point where it may have little or no effect in your body. Should we be able to do the same thing with diabetes?

No, disease suppression is not a cure, but it is very close . . .

THE REAL TRUTH ABOUT DIABETES AND WHY LIES ARE KILLING YOU

I want to make you aware of a number of myths and half-truths about diabetes. Many of these falsehoods are readily believed today even by some doctors! The truth is, few people actually know what diabetes really is, -- or there would be an accepted cure by big medicine.

Here are the myths that are perpetuating misery and suffering by helping you to maintain your disease:

- ✓ **You cannot eat sugar if you are a diabetic –** yes, you must regulate processed sugar intake but a small amount of sugar, especially from natural sources like locally grown organic honey, are actually quite good for diabetics. Moderation is key and careful timing means an occasional sweet treat will not kill you.

- ✓ **Type II diabetes is better than type I diabetes -** this myth has been perpetuated for many years. This is based on the premise that not taking insulin means that you are healthier. While physiologically this may be true, people that use insulin can readily regulate their overall blood sugar and keep it lower, thereby reducing the damage that high glucose levels do. Both types of diabetes are considered health risks.

✓ **Type II diabetes only affects fat people -** this is another myth that is untrue. Approximately 30% of people that contract type II diabetes are average weight, and the majority of people that contract type II diabetes are only moderately overweight.

✓ **People with diabetes should eat diabetic food -** nothing could be further from the truth as most types of diabetic foods **are highly processed**. They may not contain much sugar, but as you recall, it is toxic overload that keeps your body from functioning properly and makes you insulin resistant. The best foods for any diabetic to eat are 100% natural and organic whole foods, super foods and a small amount of high quality fats and honey or a pinch of cane sugar (natural) for flavor.

✓ **People with diabetes go blind and lose their legs -** while it is true that people who do not control their glucose level readings can eventually suffer from an amputation or potential blindness, all of this can be prevented by keeping your blood glucose at those levels within the realm of normal (100

- 120 to 140 or at least below 200 whenever possible).

✓ **People with diabetes are more likely to be sick -** this is also completely untrue as long as you maintain a reasonable blood glucose levels. Inflammation based on high glucose readings can lead to secondary infections, which can cause ulcers on your feet, legs etc., so maintain good sugar levels and avoid all of this.

✓ **Diabetes is contagious sometimes -** this is completely false. The only way you can contract diabetes is toxic overload of your body to the point where it can no longer regulate blood glucose levels.

✓ **Diabetics have issues driving cars -** again another crazy myth. The same rules apply to driving like they would to anyone else. As long as you have the ability to see properly and react sufficiently, diabetics are just as skilled as other drivers.

As you can see, there is a whole host of craziness that is actually believed by a majority of people who are unfamiliar with diabetes. If you hear someone repeat any of these myths, please debunk them immediately for the benefit of all of us.

DIABETES TYPE I & II AND WHAT YOU

NEED TO KNOW

Some people have a difficult time understanding the difference between type I and type II diabetes. While there are even smaller subset groups (i.e. Gestational diabetes) the real difference is based on the following factors:

- ✓ **Pre-diabetes** - this is when your body is reaching the tipping point between toxic overload and the ability to regulate blood glucose levels. Here your body is having problems processing high levels of glucose in your blood, but the readings are not yet high enough to be called type II diabetes.

- ✓ For example, normal blood glucose readings are approximately 120. Pre-diabetes usually is diagnosed when readings are between 140 -160. Even if your doctor sees elevated readings, you will typically be prescribed a drug like Metformin, which will help regulate and control sugar levels without the need for insulin.

- ✓ **Type II diabetes** - typically a diagnosis of type II diabetes results when your blood those levels are above 160 and cannot be controlled very easily through diet and exercise. Although type II diabetics are not insulin-dependent, as their pancreas is still producing some insulin, it is not in sufficient amounts. Eventually your pancreas may stop producing insulin altogether, especially if you use prescriptions.

✓ **Type I diabetes** – in this scenario type I diabetics require regular insulin shots in order to replace insulin that is not being produced by the pancreas. Continued use of insulin practically guarantees that your pancreas will never function properly because you're introducing the required insulin into the bloodstream, which prevents the restart of the pancreas.

Regardless of the actual diagnosis that you receive, dealing with both type I and type II diabetes should essentially be the same:

✓ Reduce all intake of processed junk foods and processed sugars.

✓ Stop drinking coffee, alcohol and sports drinks!

✓ Start eating only 100% organic foods that are unprocessed and have not been with any form of pesticides or contaminants.

✓ Begin detoxification of your entire body as explained in this guide later on.

✓ CONSULT WITH DOCTOR - gradually reduce your diabetic medications as your body regains its health, but always keep your blood glucose levels as close to normal as possible.

✓ Drink the cleanest water you can find - typically this is water you may need to manufacture by using proper water filtration. The water that you drink should be 100% toxin free, so find the very best water filter that removes fluorides, glyphosates, and other of dangerous and poisonous toxins. Do not drink municipal city water, do not drink bottled water, rather manufacture your own. I highly suggest looking into a Berkey water filter as this is one of the best water filters you can purchase.

I cannot emphasize enough how drinking **clean water** is absolutely essential to detoxification and recovery from most of the side effects of diabetes. Don't purchase water from the grocery store, don't buy bottled water because almost all bottled water that is sold is highly contaminated with fluoride and other minerals and toxins that are made to improve the taste, but are also highly toxic.

The goal is to completely detoxify your body so that it can recover and begin functioning normally.

MEDICAL KNOWLEDGE ABOUT DIABETES

Diabetes is a very serious medical condition that requires daily observation of blood glucose levels and then reacting to those levels by either reducing caloric intake and/or taking medications.

The medical approach to diabetes is not to try to "cure" it but rather manage the disease so that it doesn't kill you.

One of the best ways to prevent health issues from occurring is to first learn how to control your blood sugar. Controlling your blood sugar need not be overly difficult, but you must understand that proper control requires several things:

- ✓ **An understanding** of how certain foods affect your current blood glucose levels.

- ✓ **How to control your glucose levels** by moderating the food you eat and when you eat it.

- ✓ **Constantly monitoring blood glucose levels** and adjusting your medication use contingent on a sliding scale via medications you can use to counter rising sugar levels.

As most diabetics can tell you, they begin to learn exactly what happens after they consume certain foods.

For example, Joe starts out his day with a blood glucose reading of 160. Joe decides he is hungry and would still like to have breakfast so he has two eggs, two strips of bacon and one slice of toast.

An hour after Joe eats, his blood sugar rises to 256. Joe is insulin-dependent so he shoots approximately 6 units of insulin based on a sliding scale of how much he needs. An additional hour later, Joe's reading is 196, not fantastic but below 200. The next day, Joe skips the toast with breakfast and adds 12 ounces of green tea that is unsweetened.

Joe now knows exactly how to achieve a blood glucose rating of lower than 200 just by observing the food that he eats and the amounts. Joe has now "dialed in" breakfast and in the future, he knows exactly what to do to keep his blood sugar below 200.

This is the kind of information that you should **jot down in a daily journal** because the more you understand how your body reacts to certain amounts of food, the easier it will be to maintain those levels.

As you discover the right amounts of food to eat, you can begin structuring your meals so that it will be much easier to maintain proper sugar levels.

Notice that when Joe begins to add to the organic components (i.e. green tea) that his numbers begin to improve almost immediately. Eating whole foods and consuming natural teas is a great start and can be used to add more nutrients to your diet. Almost all diabetics benefit from a completely organic diet with high levels of organic teas.

MANAGE YOUR DIABETES

Since we are discussing the medical model, yes it is possible to manage your diabetes until such time as you are completely detoxified. Below are the steps that most people go through before they realize it is just managing their diabetes. I wanted to present this because the medical model does work to manage diabetes and this is the first step to controlling and eventually suppressing the disease:

- ✓ **Being diagnosed** - nothing happens in the medical world until you receive a diagnosis. While this bothers some people, being labeled a diabetic is not a death sentence unless you allow it to happen. Getting diagnosed is actually good because now you can quantify exactly what problems you are having and how you can go about correcting them.

- ✓ **Receiving the final diagnosis** - most doctors will first attempt to discern whether or not you are pre-diabetic. If you happen to be pre-diabetic, there is still hope because you are capable of preventing full-blown diabetes by making some lifestyle changes at this point. Pre-diabetes is fully curable.

This is where the false assumption is made that diabetics are simply fat, lazy and sit around all day eating sugar. In reality we now know that toxic overload is the main reason why you are receiving the diagnosis.

✓ **Welcome to the club** - Congratulations! You are now officially a diabetic. Most of us do not want to belong to the club but there are a few perks that we will discuss later.

✓ **Follow your doctor's orders** - It is at this point that your doctor will give you a selection of different medications. I strongly suggest you follow the advice at first while simultaneously following the steps in this guide.

✓ **Start following the steps in this guide.**

DIABETIC RESEARCH DETAILS

Fully understanding the most current research will give you an edge over other people suffering. The latest research also confirms everything I am teaching you here today even if modern medicine does not accept the findings yet.

I want to remind you that a majority of doctors believed less than 100 years ago **that smoking cigarettes as many as possible, was good for your lungs** and help to improve your breathing!

Always remember this example when doctors tell you they know what they're talking about . . .

Still you should follow the advice of your doctor, at least when it comes to managing diabetes. What you should not do is put your entire life in their hands. Use medical knowledge to help you manage the disease and prevent it from getting out of control.

Use the information in this guide to suppress diabetes to the point where it no longer bothers you, causes issues, or makes you ill. Always remember that modern medicine seeks only to maintain or might even worsen your diabetes because there is big money in this disease:

 "Mainstream medicine largely fails in treating diabetes – even worsens it – because it refuses to investigate and act on this underlying cause. Insulin sensitivity is key in this matter." –Dr. Mercola

Holistic practitioners like Doctor Mercola, have been sounding the alarm for many years about diabetes and other diseases that are caused predominantly by lifestyle and the toxins that we consume on a daily basis that eventually damage cells:

"According to the paper titled, "Autoimmunity against a defective ribosomal insulin gene product in type 1 diabetes," the findings "further support the emerging concept that beta cells are destroyed in T1D by a mechanism comparable to classical antitumor responses where the immune system has been trained to survey dysfunctional cells in which errors have accumulated."

Translation in simple laymen's terms: damage to cells causes other cells to attack the bad ones and this "causes" diabetes:

"New study results challenge traditional ideas about the source of type 1 diabetes (T1D). T1D, previously known as juvenile diabetes, affects an estimated 1.5 million Americans and is the result of the loss of insulin-producing cells in the pancreas. The prevailing belief was that the root cause of T1D was the immune system mistakenly identifying those insulin-secreting beta cells as a potential danger and, in turn, destroying them."

Yes it is about cell health. With T-cell research also ongoing, replacing damaged T cells is also a viable therapy that can replace insulin.

DIABETES FROM ANOTHER PERSPECTIVE

Already you may be looking at diabetes with new eyes. This is because **you finally see diabetes from a different perspective**. You now know that diabetes is a form of toxic overload to the point where your body begins to break down.

Once you know this, you're now ready to begin to explore a different way and/or different perspective on how to deal with diabetes. This will also allow you to analyze information from top experts like Dr. Richard Johnson.

Dr. Richard Johnson is most likely one of the top influential experts when it comes to fully understanding diabetes and its impact on our lives. If you are not aware, Doctor Johnson is known for his award-winning books, *The Sugar Fix* and *The Fat Switch.*

The reason why these books are so important is because they give a new insight when it comes to properly dealing with diabetes from a different perspective:

Insulin resistance - here Dr. Johnson discusses how the rise in use of high fructose corn syrup is one of the top culprits when it comes to insulin resistance.

Weight gain - high fructose corn syrup *is proven* to be the main culprit behind weight gain even if you eat a low volume of overall calories. The toxins direct the body to consume lean body mass as well. This means less muscle, more toxins, in a vicious cycle.

The reason why Dr. Johnson's work is so groundbreaking is because it follows along exactly what we are discussing here. High fructose corn syrup is an additive that is found ubiquitously in food and beverages in our society.

Were you aware that high fructose corn syrup also was processed with a form of mercury (highly toxic and considered a dangerous poison) in small amounts, enough to cause ongoing illnesses, weight gain, metabolic syndrome and a variety of other disorders and diseases?

Here is what Dr. Axe had to say and these were just some of the health issues related to high fructose corn syrup:

- Americans consume at least of 50 grams of HFCS every day.

- HFCS represents over 40 percent of caloric sweeteners added to foods and beverages.

- HFCS can increase the risk of high blood pressure, diabetes and heart disease.

➢ Consumption of HFCS has greatly increased over the years and is a main factor in our current obesity epidemic.

➢ HFCS can cause LGS or leaky gut syndrome.

➢ HFCS contains up to 570 micrograms of health-hazardous mercury per gram.

➢ HFCS has been shown to promote cancer.

➢ The average 20-ounce soda contains 15 teaspoons of sugar, all of it high fructose corn syrup.

So many doctors are now beginning to see the light especially if they do research on food additives. Obviously, what you eat is extremely important to your health and wellness. If you are consuming any high fructose corn syrup, you must eliminate it from your diet immediately. Believe me that will not be easy.

DIABETIC PRE - SUPPRESSION STARTER

I think we can all agree that we discovered the main culprit in why any of us are suffering from diabetes. *A toxic body!* So, what exactly have people done to suppress their own diabetes? Are people having success and how are they going about it?

Detoxification is our next step, and I'm going to show you exactly how to do it by drinking a series of handmade tonics from a variety of natural and organic products that are available over-the-counter. I'm referring to super foods, herbs and a combined liquid tincture that you will be able to consume (drink).

The rest of the main detoxification process is 100% contingent on your success. You must be absolutely sugar-free for at least 30 days because:

- ✓ This begins the entire detoxification process.

- ✓ This will allow your body to purge high levels of sugar and drastically drop your A1C.

- ✓ Sugar is the driving force behind elevated glucose levels so the first and fastest way to regain your health is to stop consuming it!

✓ The breakdown of toxins will slowly begin to detoxify your cells

THE DETOXIFICATION STEPS

Here I want to review the full series of steps necessary for:

✓ Pre-detoxification.

✓ Primary detoxification.

✓ Maintenance detoxification.

The steps on the following page will direct you through all of these important phases so that your body is completely clean and free of most inhibiting toxins.

The detoxification process will allow you to overlap successive steps that are progressive and gentle your body. You will build upon one level of detoxification after another.

When you have completed all the steps we will then discuss how to further push the envelope for diabetic disease suppression.

The human body has amazing potential to heal itself once the right elements are in place and the toxins are removed from your body. After a through detoxification, we will discuss how it is possible to jumpstart your pancreas and other organs.

STEP 1 – REAL WATER

Step 1: Drink ONLY purified water or created water via filtration throughout your day, as well as the purest form of Japanese green longleaf NATURAL / ORGANIC teas for your beverages.

1. **Drinking the cleanest and best form of water** possible is something that we have already discussed. You must not drink any form of municipal city water, or water from wells near farms unless filtered with a <u>Berkey water filter.</u> We suggest the Berkey brand because it is one of the few filtration systems that can remove fluoride and glyphosates from water (as well as numerous other contaminants). Do not proceed to the other steps until you are capable of producing the cleanest possible water that is as close to 100% toxin free as possible.

2. **Begin drinking water early in the morning when you first wake up on an empty stomach -** there are numerous studies that are emerging that show drinking clean water first thing in the morning *triggers toxins to flow out of your body*. However, this will ***not*** work with any type of contaminated water.

3. **Increase the amount of water that you consume until you are drinking water throughout the day -** You are attempting to flood your body with clean water and begin to push toxins out of your cells and body; so you must drink large amounts of water. Make sure that you spread the amount of water that you drink throughout the day. For example, you may wish to drink 12 ounce glasses of pure clean drinking water every 2 hours or more often if the environment is really hot.

This process begins the detoxification flush of your body. Think of it like flushing a radiator in a car. Over the period of several weeks this process will significantly help with detoxification and should be something that everyone is doing.

STEP 2 –APPLE CIDER VINEGAR

Step 2: Consume 1 tablespoon of organic apple cider vinegar daily, ½ tablespoon in the morning and ½ tablespoon at night. Apple cider vinegar may be one of the best natural and organic detoxification products on the market. It has dozens of beneficial effects:

- Apple cider vinegar gently detoxifies your body from heavy metals, foodborne toxins and other contaminants in the body.

- Apple cider vinegar can help you control high blood pressure.

- Apple cider vinegar can help you control your weight.

- Apple cider vinegar will help you maintain a natural alkalinity state.

- Apple cider vinegar will help you to regulate your blood sugar.

- Apple cider vinegar improves overall heart health.

- Apple cider vinegar can greatly reduce or eliminate Candida / fungus infections in the body.

- Apple cider vinegar reduces and controls many digestive ailments.

- Apple cider vinegar can help prevent osteoporosis.

- Apple cider vinegar greatly reduces free radical damage.

Apple cider vinegar is essentially one of the best "curatives" that you could consume on a daily basis.

Simply add half a tablespoon to 8 to 12 ounces crystal clean slightly warm water and drink it on an empty stomach in the morning and just before you go to bed at night.

Do so daily and watch your health begin to improve.

There are many other benefits of Apple cider vinegar, so make sure you do your research and always drink Apple cider vinegar directly mixed in water and never straight from the bottle as this can constrict your esophagus and throat and cause discomfort.

STEP 3 – DETOXIFY YOUR GUT

Step 3: A complete detoxification of your gut - by using one of the best products currently on the market called <u>Oxy Powder</u>.

After careful consideration of multiple products that exist, **Oxy Powder** may be the single best way to completely detoxify your gut.

If you have already been using Apple cider vinegar, you've begun this process. Oxy powder uses *oxygenation of the large and small intestine* to loosen toxins gently and naturally and then pass them out in waste.

Many other forms of gut detoxification products that are sold in stores **can have harsh side effects** and may even keep you from your daily tasks during this process.

Oxy Powder has some of the top reviews in the world and gently cleans your intestines and allows you to void (poop) all of the toxins out of your body when you visit the bathroom.

While using Oxy Powder, you can literally drop between 3 and 7 pounds of some of the most toxic waste that is been clinging to the insides of your intestines for years. You will not need to take time off from work, as long as you can make it to the bathroom several times a day! I have used this product and results were incredible.

It is well worth detoxifying your gut because this is where most health issues begin and then spread to other parts of the body. If you have a clean gut, you are much less likely to develop serious diseases and your immune system greatly improves, as well as your ability to digest nutrients.

Detoxification of your gut should be followed by an introduction of natural healthy gut bacteria, with which Apple cider vinegar also will assist. Start eating Greek yogurt, and other fermented foods to restore natural and good gut bacteria after you are done fixing your gut.

STEP 4 – GET THE BEST POSSIBLE VITAMINS

Step four: Obtain the very best possible nutraceuticals and/or vitamins that money can buy.

Part of the reason why people become diabetics is

not only due to toxic overload but also because they lack critical vitamins like magnesium. Many studies have demonstrated that high quality, natural and plant-based vitamins can have a dramatic impact on the reduction and/or suppression of diabetes.

I'm not talking about synthetic vitamins that anyone can buy over the counter. I am talking about vitamins that have been specifically created from plant extracts and that are 100% natural.

For example, the top vitamin company called Youngevity might produce some of the world's best natural supplements.

As a diabetic, it is imperative that you have proper vitamins because your body is deficient and needs these additional vitamins to effect repairs and to change the course of the disease in your body. There is simply no way to eat enough healthy food to get the benefits that you need in order to improve your health.

NOW START THE FULL SUPPRESSION PROCESS

Now that you've completed all of the detoxification processes, it's time for the suppression of your diabetes. This will completely cleanse the rest of your body, your kidneys, your pancreas, and even your liver will benefit.

The suppression process works by involving natural and organic substances that overlap each other and have a synergistic effect when it comes to jumpstarting your body and continuing to completely detoxify any remaining toxins that are preventing your body from operating correctly.

Detoxification is a process that should be ongoing, continuous and progressive. The cleaner your body is, the more efficiently it will operate. Even if you are elderly, keeping your organs clean and operating at peak efficiency can allow you to add multiple years to your life.

New research is concluding that if you can remain disease free you will be able to extend your life almost indefinitely! I'm sure you've heard stories of people living to be well past hundred years old, and you could be one of them.

Scientists have discovered that there really is no reason for us to age except when our cells break down and we eventually die if we cannot maintain healthy bodies.

Additional research is beginning to expose the importance of consuming high levels of organic material on a daily basis to extend life and prevent disease. Diabetes is a disease caused by toxic overload so the more we focus on the removing of toxins and the proper functioning of organs, the easier it will be to suppress the disease.

FULL SUPPRESSION OF DIABETES TONIC

Now that you have taken all of the steps for the pre-detoxification, it is time to move into primary detoxification.

Not only is this tonic great for your overall health, but over time you will actually grow to enjoy drinking the tonic. Essentially what the tonic will do is finish the work that was started with your pre-detoxification, which includes the following benefits:

- ✓ All of the benefits of Apple cider vinegar as mentioned earlier.

- ✓ A significant reduction of inflammation in your body, which reduces the chance of developing serious diseases.

- ✓ A complete detoxification of your liver, gallbladder and pancreas. These three organs work together synergistically in order to protect your body from disease.

- ✓ Significant improvements to digestion, hair and skin.

Here is the suggested mixture and it should be consumed each morning on an empty stomach just like the three detoxification steps. Again, it is critical that you use the cleanest possible water and 100% organic ingredients:

✓ 12 ounces of filtered warm water

✓ 1 tablespoon of raw organic liquid coconut oil

✓ ½ tablespoon of organic apple cider vinegar

✓ 1 tablespoon of organic lime juice

✓ 1 tablespoon of organic lemon juice

✓ One * pinch of Turmeric (organic / ground)

-As mentioned before, everything must be absolutely fresh!

Directions: in a cup place 12 ounces of super filtered, completely toxin free water. Squeeze half an organic line and half an organic lemon and add the juice to 12 ounces of water. Mix in turmeric (about half a teaspoon), coconut oil and stir the entire mixture.

It is important that you mix into water all the ingredients thoroughly, especially the Apple cider vinegar which never be consumed without water.

You should also make sure that you can purchase the cleanest form of turmeric which was processed here in America and not from overseas sources unless the turmeric is considered 100% pure. This is important as some forms of turmeric are polluted with small trace amounts of lead. Processing needs to be organic and natural.

MAINTENANCE TONIC . . .

After finalizing the first two stages, you can now move on to the maintenance detoxification tonic. This is slightly different because you only need to take it every other day.

The tonic now adds rosemary (a small amount), which is a super antioxidant, memory booster, and has dozens of additional health benefits. Simply adding ½ teaspoon of finely ground organic rosemary will do the trick and extend the detoxification tonic without the need to drink it every day, a real bonus when you are traveling or can't always drink the tonic:

MAINTENANCE TONIC:
- ✓ 12 ounces of filtered warm water

- ✓ 1 tablespoon of raw organic liquid coconut oil

- ✓ **½ teaspoon organic, finely ground rosemary**

- ✓ ½ tablespoon of organic apple cider vinegar

- ✓ 1 tablespoon of organic lime juice

- ✓ 1 tablespoon of organic lemon juice

- ✓ One * pinch of Turmeric (organic / ground)

The maintenance tonic is prepared the exact same

way as the main detoxification tonic. Do NOT take more than ½ a teaspoon of rosemary (a pinch) as too much can upset your stomach. One half a teaspoon seems to be enough for all the health benefits.

AT A GLANCE STEPS & TIMEFRAME FOR IT ALL

Here we are going to lay out the exact timeframe, steps and functions of the entire process to help with full understanding:

Diabetic Suppression– The suppression starter steps are the *detoxification steps* as mentioned earlier in the guide that fall under the "pre-detoxification" label:

> **Pre-detoxification** - Here you follow the first 4 steps that lead into the primary detoxification:

> **Step 1 – Real Water** – start creating and drinking over the course of the entire program.

> **Step 2 –Apple Cider Vinegar–** Start drinking over the course of the entire program.

> **Step 3 – Detoxify Your Gut** – 3-5 days, repeat twice for the first month.

- ➢ **Step 4 – Get The Best Possible Vitamins –** start taking the vitamins over the course of the entire program.

- ➢ **Primary detoxification** – take the main detoxification tonic for at least 30 days before switching to the maintenance tonic.

- ➢ **Maintenance detoxification** – switch to the maintenance tonic and drink it every other day. After 30 days, drink it every third day.

That's it! These steps are easy to follow. Simply start at the top and work your way down. Make sure that if you start having increases in blood sugar that you go back to the maintenance tonic every other day if switching to every third say has diminishing returns.

SHOPPING LIST FOR EVERYTHING YOU NEED

- ✓ **Distilled / filtered water** with NO additives of any kind OR

- ✓ **Berkey water filter** to make clean water from filtration.

- ✓ **One bottle of organic apple cider vinegar** (Braggs is the best with organic white sediment on the bottom).

- ✓ **Vitamins from a top proven plant extract based source** and do NOT buy over the counter crap from places like GNC (NO synthetic GMO laced products).

- ✓ **Organic limes** (do NOT use the processed plastic filled limes).

- ✓ **Organic lemons** (do NOT use the processed plastic filled lemons).

- ✓ **Organic coconut oil** (100% natural, virgin and liquid form).

- ✓ **Organic finely ground Turmeric**.

- ✓ **Organic and finely ground rosemary**.

When you are shopping, try to get all of your ingredients from health food stores or farmer's markets if possible. Check to make sure everything is toxin free, unprocessed and natural.

You should also locate good sources of organic foods so that you can continue to improve your health and reset your body.

Always make sure you have several clean sources for organic produce.

OTHER CONSIDERATIONS

- **Do NOT consume ANY processed sugar for at least 30 days** and significantly longer if possible. Start weaning yourself off of as much sugar as possible except natural / local honey.

- **Once your body is restored,** you will be able to eat small amounts, but always think of sugar like rat poison if you are a diabetic. Consuming as little as possible when detoxifying your body is very important.

- **ONLY use Stevia while detoxifying -** Stevia is much better than sugar as it is a plant extract. I carry a small bottle with me everywhere I go and use small amounts of it for coffee, teas etc.

- **The detoxification steps** will work in conjunction with your body. The steps are designed to complement and overlay a progressive series of cleansing actions. By following the steps, you will not shock your system or need to stop the process.

- **Watch blood sugar like a hawk–** You MUST carefully track your blood sugar especially during the entire process so that you can gradually wean yourself off of your diabetic meds. You should keep a journal and use it to show your doctor and explain what you are doing. The readings will prove to the doctor you are on the right course.

- **Reduce medication over time based on blood sugar readings at least 5 times a day**

– as your blood sugar continues to drop to normal levels you MUST wean yourself off of meds. Do NOT attempt this without your doctor. You do NOT want to have your blood sugar so low that you go into a coma.

- **Start eating super foods** for snacks. This can include blueberries, strawberries, nuts of all kinds (unsalted & skin intact), avocados, and lose leaf teas of all kinds (natural and unprocessed).

- **Soak in a hot bath daily or long hot shower** – There are many reasons to do this as a diabetic. Hot water has been the secret to longevity for people in Japan, and many studies are emerging on the benefits of daily hot water immersion.

- **Intermittent fasting** – Exciting new research is happening in this field. Intermittent fasting was part of our lifestyle as hunter/gathers for over a million (possibly longer) years or so. Our genetics cause us to NEED fasting and studies are showing that fasting up to 72 hours may completely reset our endocrine system, and heal damage in your body thought un-healable (i.e. wounds, nerves, brain cells etc.). Some diabetics are claiming that ongoing intermittent fasting "reversed" their diabetes when they resumed an organic diet after fasting. Check with your doctor, as this might not be advisable for your current condition.

- **Lose extra weight through intermittent fasting & diet change** – This should make sense. Here you start a good organic diet that is mostly plant based. Skip eating twice a week for 24 hours at least and start a low impact exercise regimen like beginner's yoga (also very good for diabetics).

- **If man made it, don't eat it** – a very simple rule to follow. If you do, your health will change for the better quickly. Stick to super foods, organic produce and grass fed, free range, no hormone meats. NEVER buy your meat from big chains (i.e. Wal-Mart) as much of their foods are tainted with toxins. Remember China now handles most of our food processing production and they have been caught doing horrible things to all foods.

Read more here:

https://offgridsurvival.com/foodsupplycontrol/

RESTORING HEALTH IS A PROCESS

Restoring health has always been a process. You do not become unhealthy overnight (usually) and steps leading up to a serious illness can be almost always prevented.

In this section we're going to discuss several ways that restoring health can be done systematically and progressively.

Unlike fad diets, quick fixes and snake oil products, here you have the opportunity to completely restore your health by relearning **what** you eat, **how** you eat and even **when** you eat.

It should make complete sense to you that something we do to our bodies **multiple times a day** (what you eat) has a dramatic impact on your overall health. The food that you take into your body must be the cleanest source possible and we have been discussing this all throughout the guide.

I want you to take the next several pages into serious consideration!

HOW TO CHANGE YOUR DIET EASILY

Unlike ridiculous fad diets, or starvation diets (this is not intermittent fasting!) Your goal is to provide your body with the proper nutrients and fuel so that it can function right and completely fight off diabetes.

One of the best ways to do this is to plan in advance how you can begin to change the number of times you are eating non-organic foods. Most people eat between four and eight times a day. We've been brought up to have breakfast, lunch, dinner and snacks.

Is this really a healthy way to eat? Absolutely not! By simply comparing our genetic memories with our ancient ancestors, let's take a look at how they typically ate food:

Breakfast - breakfast for our ancestors often consisted of berries, nuts, grains, tubers and anything else that could be harvested quickly.

Lunch – Hunter / gatherers typically did not stop for lunch and would use available daylight hours to continue to gather different types of foods to bring back to the tribe. Anything that could be found along the way may have been used for a quick snack.

Dinner -primitive man would seek out high calorie kills and bring it back to the tribe. Unfortunately, this did not happen daily and it was quite possible for people to go several days without eating large amounts of calories from protein, bone broth and marrow.

We have discovered that when we mimic the same type of hunter/ gatherer lifestyle, this induces extreme health and wellness, especially if this type of eating is coupled with occasional intense exercise.

Exercise should start out easy but become challenging.

When you compare this with the typical sedentary lifestyle of people today, is it any wonder that we are so unhealthy?

The human body was never intended to consume large quantities of sugar and doing so is equivalent to introducing a dangerous poison into your body. The typical food intake of primitive man may look something like this:

Day one – a handful of berries in the morning. Water to drink. Field greens for the afternoon and evening.

Day two – a small amount of honey followed by rabbit stew with lentils, tubers and herbs.

Day three – here the tribe has managed to get a large calorie kill so now we can add protein and high fat intake to their diet along with field greens and tubers.

Day four – the tribe is on the move today so they will only be drinking water and eating a handful of fruits and berries.

Day five - an intense storm keeps the tribe huddled in their shelters. Nobody eats today.

Day six - the tribe emerges after the storms and begins traveling to follow game. Hunters are out looking for food.

Day seven – the tribe manages another high calorie proteins kill but nobody gets to eat until later in the evening.

As you can see, primitive man ate very little, was constantly on the move and was periodically experiencing intermittent fasting. Human beings thrived on this diet and it is the modern foundation to what professionals are now calling the Paleo diet. We should be mimicking this lifestyle because we are genetically programmed to become healthy if we do so!

CONSIDER PRIMITIVE EATING TO REVERSE DIABETES

If you haven't already figured it out, primitive eating may be the best possible solution along with the steps in this guide.

You should follow all of the steps first, and as your health improves, systematically switch over to primitive eating. The goal is to follow this type of diet and/or lifestyle at least 80% of the time.

By doing so, you will guarantee that your body will continue to grow in overall fitness and health. You will use food as your primary medicine, and so you need not worry about side effects from drugs.

Ask any diabetic if that sounds like a wonderful deal, and they will tell you "absolutely." The good thing about eating primitive foods that you **do not have to be overly concerned about blood sugar**; very few super foods and or whole foods will seriously spike your blood sugar as long as they are low glycemic and you eat in moderation.

Low glycemic foods are helpful if they are whole foods and 100% natural. Never buy processed low glycemic diet foods, as yet again they are filled with toxins.

Also, you should consider going from the current diet you were eating to a primitive diet over time. You should never completely quit cold turkey the food you are eating, but rather slowly and gradually replace high calorie, high carbohydrate processed foods for the better food choices.

Finally, if you have any doubts as to whether or not primitive eating is good for you, tens of thousands of people have switched to this type of lifestyle and many of them are reporting vibrant health, increased physical strength and stamina and other health benefits that are essentially too numerous to list here. Maybe it's time for you to consider primitive eating to reverse your diabetes.

WHAT TO EXPECT IN 90 DAYS ON THIS PROGRAM

Once you have followed all the steps in this guide, you should begin to see blood sugar readings drop considerably.

You will also experience other physiological and even psychological changes; so I wanted to make a list of these for you so that you are not surprised and can anticipate what will happen to you:

- ➢ **Consistent and downward blood glucose readings** from high to manageable (i.e. 250 to 190). Remember it takes time for your body to heal, so the reduction will be gradual will also be based on the kind of diet you are eating.

- ➢ **Greatly reduced cravings for sugar** - essentially sugar to a diabetic is like crack cocaine to a drug abuser. By completely weaning yourself off of processed sugars, you will notice that you will begin to feel better almost immediately and that over time, cravings will gradually lessen.

- ➢ **Improve mental clarity and focus** - When you're eating the correct foods, mind and body begin to work well together. A mental fog that follows most diabetics begins to lift and you will notice being able to think more clearly and make better decisions.

> **A gradual reduction to possible complete elimination of all diabetic drugs -** The idea is to gradually wean yourself off of these drugs as well because they are only maintaining your disease and not curing it.

> **Improved skin tone, shiny hair, bright eyes** – additional awesome benefits of following all the steps in this guide.

> **A vibrant look of health and wellness -** as your health continues to prove, and your body is finally working correctly, you will begin to exude health and have a general appearance of someone who is radiant and well.

> **Weight loss without dieting -** By following all the steps in this guide you'll naturally lose weight because you'll be eating the correct foods. Some people become concerned because you will tend to drop a significant amount of weight; but this is natural and is a form of detoxification in and of itself.

> **Reduced depression -** Eating the correct balance of nutrients is more effective than any prescription drug for depression. When you're getting the correct balance of

nutrients your mind is in balance with your body.

> **Improved sleeping patterns** - Eating the right food and keeping your diabetes suppressed means that we are able to have much more productive sleep, which will continue to improve our health as well. Diabetics need at least eight hours of uninterrupted sleep and good sleeping patterns.

> **Improved digestion** - A majority of digestive issues, such as Crohn's disease, are caused by eating junk foods. Switching to whole foods and primitive eating can cure all digestive issues over time because your body has time to heal and regenerate.

> **Stable and easily maintained blood sugar levels** – the result of all of this for a diabetic is near normal blood sugar levels.

These are all fantastic reasons why following the steps in this guide can truly benefit you.

Now you completely understand how to repair almost all damage to your body, by simply following primitive eating.

HOW IT ALL WORKED FOR "RALPH"

One man by the name of **Ralph** was following the advice in this guide. He informed his doctor that he was attempting to utilize natural methods to help control his blood sugar.

I wanted to include Ralph's story because he was a typical person who was diabetic and he is proof that this system works.

Ralph lived in Upstate New York and was a father of two boys. About ten years ago he began to notice he felt tired and lethargic. Over time, it was discovered that he was having issues controlling his blood sugar.

Like most people, we listen to our doctor at first. When Ralph visited his physician, he was told that according to the blood tests, he was most likely pre -diabetic.

As you recall from earlier parts of the guide, we explain what happens to people when they first receive their diagnosis and Ralph was no different.

Ralph began taking prescription drugs, which were supposed to regulate his blood sugar and help him. This principal medication was Metformin. Unknown to Ralph, side effects of this prescription drug include constipation, diarrhea, headaches, dizziness and of course reduced blood sugar.

It's interesting to note that the drug also reduces the level of vitamin B12 in the body, which is a critical nutrient. It is absolutely necessary for the health and well-being of all people, especially diabetics!

While his diabetic symptoms began to subside, he noticed that after about a year on prescription drugs that his diabetes was actually getting worse and he needed more medication to achieve the same maintenance results.

Ralph hated being on the medication but he figured he had no choice and this was just something he had to endure.

After Ralph's second year of being a diabetic he began to notice that he was having issues with his kidneys and pancreas. It was at this point that the doctor suggested adding insulin, because it would be easier for Ralph to control (maintain) this disease.

It was at this point that Ralph started taking regular shots of insulin in order to further control his diabetes, which was slowly becoming uncontrollable. Even with insulin, Ralph would occasionally have high blood sugar glucose readings, sometimes as high as 400 . . .

Of course, the insulin would always reduce his blood sugar to manageable levels, but what was really happening in his body **was that all of his organs were beginning to shut down.**

While insulin is a godsend to people and can extend their lives, it actually teaches your body not to function properly. Because of this, Ralph began searching the Internet for people who claimed that it was possible to at least control if not outright repress their own diabetes.

Ralph discovered this guide and began to apply its teachings.

At first it was difficult for Ralph, but he began to realize that diabetes was not necessarily his fault, and that all the food he believed was edible was actually filled with toxins; the primary reason why Ralph contracted diabetes in the first place.

Ralph began to follow the steps to detoxify his body so that it would begin to function normally. He stayed on all of the detoxification tonics and over a period of approximately 60 days, he saw his blood sugar finally improve dramatically.

Ralph then switched to eating almost purely organic foods, and over a period of another 30 days, saw dramatic increases in his overall health and wellness.

Ralph was very excited by the results because he was slowly reducing his medication while increasing primitive eating and using the steps in this guide to detoxify his body. What was truly amazing about the entire process is that it was actually cheaper for Ralph to follow the steps in this guide than to maintain his diabetes using expensive drugs that had horrible side effects and were not healing his body.

Ralph began to increase exercise once he regained some of his strength. First, he started out with yoga because it was very low impact and he could do this exercise at his own pace.

Ralph became quite the expert and when combining meditation and breathing exercises, his stress greatly reduced which also benefited his health. Ralph began to see real improvements and his stamina increased exponentially.

Once Ralph added intermittent fasting and primitive eating, his body was completely healed, and even though doctors say can never cure diabetes, he proved them all wrong.

Ralph reverses diabetes and so can you.

The steps in this guide are not difficult to do, are not expensive and have a huge track record of success helping and healing diabetics. What do you have to lose except the disease? And that is something all of us are very grateful to do.

HOW TO CONVINCE YOUR DOCTOR TO WORK WITH YOU

This is one of the last sections in this e-book, but one of the most important. I would like to give you some basic background information about doctors and why it isn't working to try and find the right type of doctor who will work with you while you are going through this process.

The first thing you need to know is that doctors today do not receive the same kind of training they did years ago. Nutrition is barely discussed nor are alternative healing methods.

The pharmaceutical companies make hundreds of billions of dollars off of diabetes so they are protecting their cash cow. They do so by **suppressing research**, publishing misleading information and funding most of the training that doctors receive today.

The typical doctor who goes to med school has almost all of their expenses supported by large pharmaceutical companies, who incidentally are creating and writing a fair amount of the coursework the doctors are receiving. It is all about writing prescriptions now.

Since **ongoing education is also required** to continue to practice medicine, pharmaceutical companies hold paid training for many doctors in exotic places. Most doctors simply need to sign an attendance sheet and then go enjoy a five star hotel and scenic places where many of these conferences are held.

The ongoing education consists of a variety of drugs that can be used and the latest drugs that will be coming on the market. Many doctors receive financial incentives not only to promote the drugs, but to actually prescribe them even if they are clueless as to what is really capable of doing to the human body.

The bottom line is simple: the drug companies control our doctors by providing them many of the benefits that they already should be receiving for being a good doctor.

Another huge consideration is that the primary training the doctors receive is simply inadequate and has nothing to do with curing disease or holistic medicine.

Yet we've seen the results of holistic medicine, and it is quite capable of providing different levels of disease repression or in some cases out right curatives.

By understanding all of this information, you realize that doctors are essentially "drug pushers" unless they happen to fall outside of the typical norm. For example, holistic doctors study natural ways to heal the human body and are very much interested in natural ways to do so.

You should also consider that your doctor may know absolutely nothing about the origins of diabetes. Typically, most doctors will blame diabetes **on the person who has it;** but as you can see, many of us can contract diabetes simply by interacting with our environment.

While all of us are required to eat healthy in order to stay healthy, it simply is ludicrous to blame the diabetic when there are so many smoking guns for diabetes that have been linked to a toxic environment.

With all of this understood, now you have a new way to think about how to approach your doctor. The very first step may be to find the correct doctor in the first place!

For example, remember Ralph? His doctor only wanted to prescribe medications for him and didn't want to hear anything about a so-called "folk cure." The doctor even warned Ralph not to attempt this as he might injure his health further. This is exactly what doctors are taught and why you must consider finding one that does NOT follow this thinking.

Yes, there are a large number of highly qualified

doctors that may know exactly what you're attempting to do because they focus their practice on holistic medicine.

So, the best way to involve your doctor in the first place is to consider finding the right doctor who will listen to what you have to say and already practices most of what you're trying to do.

Here is what I suggest you do to find the closest holistic doctor who will support what you want to do with your health:

- ➢ **Look online for a doctor who believes in holistic medicine** and working with patients who want to take advantage of it.

- ➢ **Find other diabetics who are like-minded** and ask them about how they handled their doctor.

- ➢ **Invest in a good journal and track your blood sugar** and foods you eat. This is valuable empirical information for any doctor and can prove that what you are doing works.

- ➢ **Never go to a general practitioner** unless you can see their track record of treating diabetes.

- ➢ **Follow all the latest research** as several breakthroughs are about to happen. For example, India has recently claimed they have a new shot that eliminates diabetes.

> **Show your doctor your progress** in your journal as this helps convince him or her that you know what you are talking about.

> **Ask about any complications** with medication. Typically there are not any, but always ask.

Many doctors are also willing to listen to you because their main job is to be like a detective; what works to make you better usually will be supported by most doctors, as long as you can prove you are getting better.

Always remember that a doctor's primary concern is the ability for them to generate sufficient income to keep their practice doors open. Due to the high cost of medical malpractice and other expenses, most doctors are willing to sell their ideals in exchange for regular income, the kind that comes with writing prescriptions all the time.

The only person that's truly going to be 100% in favor of everything you do to improve your health will be *you*. Most doctors are motivated by money, power and prestige.

Even though most people get into medicine for all the right reasons, anyone that has worked in the field will tell you that it is very corrupt and its focus is not always the patient's best interests. Doctors are routinely paid for delivering vaccines and prescriptions especially with the latest drugs they're constantly being flooded on the market.

We've seen the results of bad drugs, and as long as there are doctors pushing these drugs on unsuspecting hapless victims, medicine is no longer going to be primarily about curing anyone.

That's what happened to medicine today thanks to greedy politicians, greedy drug companies and everyone else in between who makes 'a cut' off of your poor health.

Find the right doctor in the first place if at all possible!

FIND SUPPORT GROUPS

One of the final bits of information I wish to offer to you is to consider finding the very best support groups out there.

If you can't find a support group, maybe you should start one in your area. Support groups can do many things to help everyone benefit:

- ✓ **Friends** - People who are going through the exact same thing you are may have found creative ways to deal with the disease that can help you too. You will make good friends and you may be able to help each other when diabetes becomes too much to handle by yourself.

- ✓ **Support** - Not only can you make good friends, but the main purpose of this support group is to assist you in dealing with whatever issue that group is about. There may be information that you are unaware of that could completely change the situation for you for the better. Being able to meet with other people who suffer from the same disease means that you can exchange notes and ideas on how to make yourself better.

- ✓ **Networking** - Another bonus of being part of a support group is that many different types of helpful solutions may be readily available and proven to work by other members. If one member has discovered something that makes their life easier, they can share this information with everybody else. Networking is always a benefit of joining any support group.

- ✓ **Exercise and activities** - Diabetics know they must exercise to maintain health and what a fun way to do it -- with other people whom also understand this mandate. It is far better to join in with like-minded people than to try to exercise on your own with people that are not diabetic. You will not only enjoy the group activity but you get much needed exercise.

✓ **Financial support** - Many support groups have funding and grants from businesses, entrepreneurs and philanthropists. There is money available to help you when you really need it, especially if you're a contributing member of the group on a regular basis.

✓ **Adult daycare / sitting services** - Support groups also offer ways to help others who are going through a difficult time. For example, as a new member you might be required twice a month to make yourself available for eight hours so that you can do chores, help other adults that are suffering as well as share the load when it comes to disease management.

✓ **Innovation, new research and testing** - Support groups also offer the ability to be involved in the latest diabetic research and testing of new products. While nobody likes being a guinea pig, you might just stumble across something very useful that truly improves your health and wellness.

✓ **Safety and security** – Having the ability to network with other people that are suffering with the same disease means that you can count on these people to help you when you have issues pertaining to your safety and security. For example, it is discovered that a particular diabetic medicine is causing premature death, but the information is suppressed. You are much more likely to learn this information and have it revealed to you when many people come together and pool their collective knowledge.

Support groups can also be created by going to https://www.meetup.com/. Millions of people create meet ups and diabetic\s are no exception. This is also a great way to meet like-minded people if you appreciate certain hobbies, events etc.

Why not take the time to create your own group? You could help literally hundreds maybe even thousands of people who are diabetic and that's a whole lot of positive karma coming in your direction. At your next opportunity make sure you either find or create a perfect meet up group.

CONCLUSION AND BEYOND

I wanted to first take the time to say thank you for reading this amazing guide. I have devoted a considerable amount of time to the research as well as finally explaining to people *exactly what diabetes really is* and not just what we are spoon fed from modern medicine and large pharmaceutical companies.

In this guide we discussed many controversial topics like: why hasn't there been a medical cure for diabetes released? We further explain the exact medical definition of what we are told diabetes is *should be* according to modern medicine. Boy, are they wrong!

I reveal a completely different definition of what diabetes is based on **years of research and having been a diabetic**. I explain how toxic overload eventually leads to dysfunction in the body and *smoldering illnesses* such as diabetes, which are caused by out-of-control inflammation by toxins.

I next go into exactly what junk food does to you. This includes all of the other forms of toxins that we are absorbing on a daily basis.

Most people are not aware of this.

In addition, I go into detail about the real truth and the numerous lies and disinformation that exist about the disease, which most people believe, but are untrue.

I also discussed exactly what diabetes type I and type II are as well as good information on controlling the disease.

Next, I discussed some of the better ways of diabetic management and **some of the latest diabetic research details**.

I also discussed diabetes from another perspective and how it is possible **to begin suppression of the disease** by changing what you eat and utilizing organic herbs and super foods in combination to completely suppress the disease over time.

Also, I lay out exact steps and give you several recipes for diabetic suppression tinctures that you can drink on a regular basis which are cheap, healthy, have no side effects and are easy to make.

I also explain what to do **in the maintenance stage** after you have your disease under control so that it never comes back.

Finally, I give you detailed information including 'at a glance' steps and timelines bringing everything together on a single page; so that you completely understand how the process should be followed.

Next, I explore the process of restoring your health and how you can change your diet progressively over time so that it is not a system shock when you start changing foods and eating really healthy.

I also talk about **primitive eating** and how this will affect you and your health over the next 90 days.

Finally, I bring everything together with a story about **Ralph** and the best steps for convincing your doctor to work with you. This includes finding support groups and we've explained exactly how you can do just that, even if you want to be the one who starts the support group.

I have distilled literally years of information on how to reverse diabetes based on solid research, evidence, proof and direct information that you can immediately begin to use to reverse your own diabetes.

All the information is now at your fingertips and all you have to do to systematically, gently and effectively reduce your diabetes is to follow the steps.

Now you have the solution you've been looking for and all you have to do is use this guide.

I'd like to take the opportunity to say thank you and congratulate you from the bottom of my heart for finishing this book. The next step is to implement what you have learned.

Best Regards,
David F. Wilson

MANUSCRIPT - 2

THE KETO COOKBOOK

DISCLAIMER

The author has made every attempt to be as accurate and complete as possible in the creation of this publication/PDF, however he does **not warrant or represent at any time that the contents within are accurate due to the rapidly changing nature of the Internet**. The author assumes no responsibility for errors, omissions, or contrary interpretation of the subject matter herein. Any perceived slights of specific persons, people, or organizations other published materials are unintentional and used for educational purposes only.

This information is not intended for use as a source of legal, business, accounting or financial advice. All readers are advised **to seek services of competent professionals in the legal, business, accounting, health, dietary and finance field.** No representation is made or implied that the reader will do as well from using the suggested techniques, strategies, methods, systems, or ideas as from using any others; rather it is presented for news value only.

The author does not assume any responsibility or liability **whatsoever** for what you choose to do with this information. Use your own judgment. Consult appropriate professionals before starting a business or making ANY investment. Any perceived remark, comment or use of organizations, persons mentioned or any resemblance to characters living, dead or otherwise, real or fictitious, does not mean that they support this content in any way, but is provided for news value / information only.

There are no guarantees of accuracies, diet information or health benefits. Readers are asked to consult their doctor and other medical professionals before changing their diet or consuming any foods based on this guide.

Readers are cautioned to rely on their own judgment about their individual circumstances to act accordingly. By reading any document, the reader agrees that under no circumstances is the author responsible for any losses, direct or indirect, that are incurred as a result of use of the information contained within this document, including - but not limited to errors, omissions, or inaccuracies.

INTRODUCTION - OVERVIEW

The ketogenic diet (often referred to as the *Keto diet* or *Keto lifestyle*) has been massively improving health and transforming lives for the better for millions of people every day.

The Keto lifestyle (eating & living Keto), which includes this "cookbook" is well known as first and foremost, a low carb diet but in reality, it is much more a ***lifestyle change*** from modern destructive eating habits.

With the ***Keto lifestyle***, you follow what looks like essentially a low carb way to eat. Yet instead of fueling your body with glucose (sugar), which is very destructive to your health, you also eat a majority of healthy fats and moderate proteins, and this makes your body diminish and eliminate your addiction to sugar.

Further, the Keto lifestyle begins to transform your body to run on healthy fats, <u>producing ketones</u> from your liver.

This is a godsend for **Diabetics and obese** people who should be almost eliminating all forms of sugar from their diet.

In addition, fueling your body on high natural fats, you reduce insulin and sugar issues and this begins to heal your body. All of the recipes in this cookbook are focused on this goal.

<u>Sugar is very toxic</u> even to non-diabetics and your body actually cannot handle more than a few teaspoons of processed sugar a day. The extra is converted into toxins that impact your health and eventually shorten life and the quality of life.

By eating a diet low in carbs (yes you need to eat some), the body creates a condition called **Ketosis**; this process is designed to convert fat in the liver into energy.

Primitive man was almost always in a state of Ketosis and because of it he (and she) experienced vibrant health.

The goal of a properly maintained Keto lifestyle is to force your body to remain in this state. This is NOT accomplished via starvation but rather a shift to eating the right mix of foods: about 70% healthy fats, 25% proteins and 5% carbs.

This can be achieved with 99% of the recipes herein.

There have been decades of research and experimentation, and the Keto diet was originally created to treat epilepsy and similar neurological conditions (removal of sugar cures many health issues).

Some of the **health benefits of the Keto lifestyle** include:

- ✓ Steady and ongoing fat Loss.

- ✓ Weight control even if you are obese (over time).

- ✓ Improved HDL /LDL numbers.

- ✓ Almost complete elimination of out of control blood sugar (Diabetics pay attention here).

- ✓ Insulin leveling and control.

- ✓ Increases in muscle mass.

- ✓ Energy levels skyrocketing.

- ✓ Mental focus and clarity.

- ✓ Decreased cravings and reduced hunger.

- ✓ Reduced markers for Cancer, heart disease.

If these reasons are not good enough for you to try the Keto lifestyle, then the ease of these recipes, the flavors and the quick preparation will win you over. Finally, you hold in your hands an incredible tool to completely transform your health and wellness.

Best Regards,

David F. Wilson

SECTION I: WHY YOU NEED THE KETOGENIC LIFESTYLE

"The Keytogenic lifestyle" has been said to be perhaps one of the best ways to regain control of your overall health and wellness.

The Keto lifestyle may also be **one of the best ways for accomplishing weight loss,** especially if you have tried other diets but failed.

Originally created as a way to help control epilepsy, it was discovered to be beneficial also for people who should not eat large amounts of sugar in their diets.

Multiple medical studies (over 25 to date) completely support the theory that the Keto diet / lifestyle taps into early genetic markers that work in concert with your body.

Fueling your body with healthy fats instead of sugar was how our earliest ancestors not only survived, but thrived.

Early man (and woman too) was much more physically fit, healthy, lean and strong. Some of our earliest ancestors were said to be at least twice if not three times stronger than our modern counterparts today.

Early man could run for sometimes hours without getting winded, climb trees like monkeys and were adept hunters and gatherers.

In fact, there is plenty of personal evidence that diets consisting predominately of healthy fats, moderate proteins and low carbs are the hallmark of excellent health.

Adopting the Keto lifestyle and utilizing this special master cookbook you really will begin to enjoy some amazing benefits:

Lose mostly fat stores, not lean muscle – Early man was a powerhouse of muscle and power. He or she was kept naturally slender because the ketones used for fuel were part of what fueled real health.

Think about it for a moment: over a million years of evolution came to shape our eating habits. Paleo man would go sometimes a day or two on low carbs and then eat massive amounts of natural fat laden meats.

Manage and improve heart disease - Fats were at the center of this diet for primitive man. Natural (NOT manmade) fats actually heal your heart and can restore cardiovascular health because your body needs them to run properly.

It is only with the advent of modern diets that

disease began to explode. Despite the claims made by modern medicine, we are vastly unhealthier compared to our ancestors and real disease is an extension of our modern love for sugar and contaminated pseudo foods that are foisted on us by our society. Fast foods should be called 'death foods' because study after study links processed foods as a precursor to many forms of disease including Diabetes.

Treat cancers of all kinds – The main fuel for cancer, which is very much like a fungus in the body, is sugar. Many studies link a return to natural foods like green teas, large amounts of vitamin C and cannabis oil as curatives, as long as you are completely off of all processed sugars.

The Keto lifestyle - is so effective at helping to improve lives that many diet companies are actually paying bloggers to scare people away from trying it.

Many articles are emerging warning of the dangers, but when you trace the funding back to who is actually publishing these articles, it is almost always big Agribusiness (Agra).

While you must take into consideration your medical condition before attempting any new way of eating, remember that there are lots of big players who have a vested interest in where you spend your money:

- ✓ Big Agra

- ✓ Big Pharma

- ✓ The diet industry

- ✓ The snack industry

- ✓ The medical profession

This is just to name a few. It is your body and your life. Think very carefully what you want to do before you give it to any of these corporations that do not care about you, but care very much that you eat their "franken foods," take their drugs and eat their toxic laden products. . .

SECTION II: MORE AMAZING FACTS ABOUT THE KETO DIET & WHY IT WORKS BETTER THAN ALMOST ANY OTHER "DIET"

The diet can also treat / improve many modern illnesses in addition to what we have already discussed:

Alzheimer's – There is new research finding that the coconut oil used in the diet (in many foods if you follow this cookbook) has a powerful impact on the disease and can lessen or even suppress the disease. Use of raw organic coconut oil as an additive to meals is an additional benefit.

Epilepsy / seizures - The ketogenic diet has been clinically proven to slow or even halt seizures. This is a godsend to people who suffer from seizure disorders. This also includes Parkinson's disease and other related motor function issues.

Diabetes – As mentioned before, as a diabetic you need to remove as much sugar from your diet as possible. Running your body on healthy fats and low carbs will suppress the disease to a point where it essentially no longer causes harm to your body. With Diabetes exploding across the world in massive numbers, the Keto lifestyle is one of the best options as a pre-diabetic (will cure this) or a type I or II sufferer.

Fad Diets – Almost no fad diet is good for your health and in the long run can cost you lean muscle mass. You think you are losing weight, but retaining lean muscle mass is very important especially for older people. Most fad diets strip your body of muscle mass. In addition, a vast majority of people who go on these 'yo yo' diets end up slowing their metabolism to a snail's crawl so as soon as you resume eating even partially like you used to, you pack on even more fat as your body reacts to "starvation" to protect itself from another round of fad dieting.

What does science say? **The Keto lifestyle** flies in the face of traditional diets as they are flawed:

"Some believe that increased fat in the diet is a leading cause of all kinds of health problems, especially heart disease. This is the position maintained by most mainstream health organizations. These organizations generally recommend that people restrict dietary fat to less than 30% of total calories (a low-fat diet).

However, in the past 11 years, an increasing number of studies have been challenging the low-fat dietary approach. *Many health professionals now believe that a low-carb diet (higher in fat and protein) is a much better option* to treat obesity and other chronic, Western diseases."

Source: https://authoritynutrition.com/23-studies-on-low-carb-and-low-fat-diets/

There are many studies that now reflect this very statement. People are realizing they have been sold a pack of lies designed to keep them on the diet – a junk food rollercoaster for the profits of the big corporations.

SECTION III: HOW & WHY IT WORKS, SIDE EFFECTS AND PRECAUTIONS

Understanding the benefits of the Keto Lifestyle is just part of the picture. We need to review critical information on what makes the Keto lifestyle really work and of course what can derail your progress or even potentially cause you harm.

First of all, understand what you are doing to your body when you start to follow this cookbook and the Keto way of eating:

"Ketosis occurs when people eat a low- or no-carb diet and molecules called ketones build up in their bloodstream. Low carbohydrate levels cause blood sugar levels to drop and the body begins breaking down fat to use as energy. Ketosis is actually a mild form of ketoacidosis."

Source: http://www.healthline.com/health-news/keto-diet-is-gaining-popularity-but-is-it-safe-121914

The Keto diet initially was created by a brilliant Italian doctor called **Gianfranco Cappello**, an associate professor of surgery at the Sapienza University in Italy (Rome).

The mainstream medical community was in denial

for many years concerning his research. It has taken years of irrefutable documented proof in the form of peer-reviewed white papers to finally shut up the medical community, which is now beginning to follow and recreate some of his research.

If you are diabetic or have issues with your blood sugar, the health damage you sustain must be halted at all costs.

Switching to the **Keto Lifestyle** should always be accompanied by a visit to your current physician, but always keep in mind: doctors today receive almost NO education in nutrition and are trained to write prescriptions.

It is in the best interest of big pharmaceutical companies to keep people like you sick.

PRECAUTIONS & SIDE EFFECTS

There is no perfect "diet." In fact, depriving yourself of food you want to eat causes psychological stressors that lead to depression. What you need to do is to finally understand how to **fall in love with real whole foods** and eat like your ancestors did.

When you first start the Keto Lifestyle, remember you are essentially "detoxing" from the crap foods you have been eating. This is why you should gradually ease into the lifestyle by substitution of each meal over time. For example, start eating Keto breakfasts for a week. Then add Keto snacks for a week. Finally add dinner meals.

Even if you do this carefully, shifting from a mostly sugar diet (which is very toxic) is like a drug abuser getting over his or her addiction. Never go "cold turkey" and switch 100% to Keto eating right away; **take it in steps**. If you are on medications, you must remember eating this way will heal your body over time and you may not need them anymore.

Diabetics who switch to this way of eating will no longer need insulin, or at least not in the amounts they did before.

This is why you MUST include a physician in the

plan to help you. Watch your blood sugar like a hawk and do not use the sliding scale unless approved by a doctor. Eat FIRST, wait one hour and check blood sugar again to make sure how much insulin you need, and when on the Keto diet, NEVER take insulin first.

Remember **the elimination of sugar in your diet** will reduce all kinds of health issues, including excess weight and higher blood sugar, so you may no longer need your meds, or at least not as much, so watch this carefully and with the help of a physician.

Ketogenic diet will help you lose weight and begin feeling better both physically and mentally. This keto **diet can even reverse some weight-related damage** to your body as your metabolism changes and you begin to utilize ketones for energy rather than using glucose.

Side effects of eating Keto:

1. **Keto "flu"** –Just like an addict, you need time to detox from sugar. The effects are similar but much milder; loss of appetite, some nausea, reduced energy, and reduced performance for exercise, mild digestive issues and mild sleep disorders. This will pass in about a week and some people experience no side effects if they ease into the Keto lifestyle.

2. **Sluggishness** – This is part of the "Keto Flu" and it can be countered with high quality mineral supplementation. ONLY get vitamins that are organic and derived from plant extracts, NOT synthetic. It is very important you do this because you still need plant minerals for optimum health. Try to get top supplements that top athletes use, NOT over the counter crap sold at most big chain stores, i.e. Youngevity.

3. **Exercise issues** – as you adjust to your new lifestyle remember to keep exercising, but reduce it to just the bare minimum, like walking. This gives your body time to adjust and allows you to regain strength and stamina over time.

Try to follow these suggestions, as they will help you quickly adapt and recover. Over the weeks your strength will not only return but you will begin to feel healthier than ever before.

Now that you understand everything you need to know about the Keto Lifestyle, congratulations!

We are now going to explore some of the best meals you can make quickly. Many of our recipes in this amazing cookbook are easy to prepare and can be made from some of the most common and easy to acquire foods available at your local grocery store.

Always try to get the most organic versions of the ingredients listed and avoid GMO versions. Remember part of the Keto Lifestyle is to detox naturally, so avoid any and all processed foods. Let's get started with really awesome breakfasts, then lunch/dinners and snacks. Enjoy...

KETO RECIPES TO START THE DAY: BREAKFAST / BRUNCH

Breakfast when eating a Keto diet, is a much more balanced way to start the day. Over the next thirty recipes, we will explore some of the very best dishes that both Keto dieticians and experts have been using with their students.

The foods chosen were done with several things in mind:

- ✓ **Ease of preparation** with easy to get ingredients.

- ✓ **Make most recipes** in less than 5 minutes.

- ✓ **Healthy** and affordable ingredients.

It is important to buy the best natural sources of organic, free range and hormone / pesticide free food sources from places like farmer's markets, co-ops and or whole food distributors. Try to avoid big chain stores and focus on locally produced foods.

1. "MONSTER" KETO OMELET WITH AVOCADOS

This powerhouse breakfast will not only amaze your taste buds, it is a 'quick build.' Try spice variants like garlic and you will love this great start to the day:

Ingredients:

- ✓ 3 large eggs, whisked together with a dash of salt and pepper
- ✓ 1 diced green pepper
- ✓ ½ sliced avocado, cut in thin strips
- ✓ 2 slices organic bacon, cooked & crumbled
- ✓ ½ small red onion thoroughly diced
- ✓ 1 cup fresh baby spinach
- ✓ 2 tablespoons of avocado oil
- ✓ ¼ cup mild cheddar cheese
- ✓ ¼ cup sour cream
- ✓ Optional spices like garlic, turmeric, basil

Directions:

In a small saucepan, combine one tablespoon of avocado oil with the diced greens, crumbled bacon, sour cream, spinach leaves, and onion. Cook for 2 minutes on a medium heat and remove it from the heat.

In an egg pan (small non-stick fry pan for eggs) add one tablespoon avocado oil. Add eggs in whisked form. Cook on a medium low heat until eggs solidify. Flip and cook on the other side.

Place omelet round on a plate and add the cheddar cheese. Now add all the remaining ingredients to one side of the omelet round. Fold over and garnish with remaining cheese and avocado slices. This delicious omelet will fill you up for most of the day!

2. COCONUT EGG SCRAMBLE WITH ROSEMARY & THYME

No, this is not a song lyric ("parsley, sage rosemary & thyme"), but when you are finished eating this scramble, you just might feel like singing! The coconut oil and the herbs make this a delicious morning scramble to eat on the fly. Try all of these same ingredients in a low carb veggie wrap to make the meal portable.

Ingredients:

- ✓ 3 eggs, whisked and a dash of salt and pepper added

- ✓ 2 tablespoons grass fed butter

- ✓ 2 tablespoons coconut oil

- ✓ 1 teaspoon rosemary

- ✓ 1 teaspoon thyme

- ✓ ¼ cup diced organic bacon

- ✓ ½ cup diced kale or spinach leaves

- ✓ ¼ cup organic feta cheese

- ✓ 2 veggie wraps

Directions:

In a medium fry pan, combine all ingredients

except the feta cheese and the wraps and cook on a medium heat, folding the mix.

As the scramble reduces, fold at a steady speed.

Add the finished mix to a plate and add the feta cheese.

You can also make two wraps out of the ingredients, splitting the feta cheese between the wraps and dividing the ingredients evenly.

3. SWEET & SASSY KETO BREAKFAST PORK PATTIES

If you like breakfast patties, this is a great option because you make them yourself. This will also be used in later recipes (as an option). Try these delicious patties but make sure you use free range pork.

Ingredients:

- ✓ 2 pounds pork, free range
- ✓ 1 lime, fresh squeezed
- ✓ 1 teaspoon sage
- ✓ ½ cup coconut oil
- ✓ 1 teaspoon Stevia (plant extract, sweetener, natural)
- ✓ 1 teaspoon maple extract
- ✓ dash of cayenne pepper
- ✓ salt and pepper to taste (several dashes)

Directions:

In a large prep bowl, place the pork and let stand for 30 minutes with the juice of one lime. Mix and let stand.

Now add all the other ingredients and mix thoroughly.

Preheat oven to 350 degrees. Make round patties from the ingredients, about a 3" diameter (small hockey puck size).

The recipe makes about 6-8 patties. They are flavorful and tangy as well as a healthy version of Keto meat.

4. KETO ZUCCHINI & COCONUT FLAKED SCRAMBLED EGGS

This delicious and savory variant of a classic breakfast will have you eating your veggies and loving them. Best of all, they are low carbs; just what you would expect from a brilliant Keto lifestyle.

Ingredients:

- ✓ 3 eggs, whisked together with salt and pepper (dash of each)

- ✓ 1 medium zucchini, finely diced (small cubes ¼ inch is best)

- ✓ 2 slices of crumbled organic bacon

- ✓ ½ small white onion

- ✓ 1 clove garlic, diced

- ✓ ½ cup organic coconut flakes

- ✓ 2 tablespoons coconut oil

- ✓ 1 tbsp freshly chopped parsley

Directions:

In a medium frypan, add both tablespoons of coconut oil, the clove of garlic, the onion and the zucchini. Cook on a low heat until the veggies soften, about 2-3 minutes.

Now add the eggs and scramble on a low heat for 5 minutes or until the eggs are cooked.

Add the remaining ingredients for an additional 1 minute.

One variant is to add the coconut flakes last after everything else is cooked with a touch of maple syrup extract.

5. AVOCADO BARBECUE BREAKFAST SALMON WITH EGGS

Fish, especially salmon is very good for you. Make sure you source quality wild salmon from places like Alaska, and not farm raised from large chain stores. This dish is a good alternative for brunch while still holding onto eggs for a splash of breakfast taste.

Ingredients:

- ✓ 3 eggs, free range if possible
- ✓ ½ avocado, sliced in strips
- ✓ 2 fillets of salmon medium size
- ✓ 2 tablespoons full fat cream cheese
- ✓ 2 tablespoons of coconut oil
- ✓ 2 tablespoons chopped chives
- ✓ 1 medium spring onion
- ✓ 2 teaspoons butter (organic, real butter only)
- ✓ dash of salt and pepper
- ✓ 1 cup spinach leaves
- ✓ 1 cup grated parmesan cheese

✓ 2 teaspoons barbecue seasoning

Directions:

Heat skillet on medium heat, salt and pepper thawed fillets and place on skillet with two tablespoons of coconut oil. Cook on one side until firm and sprinkle the barbecue seasoning on the fish and cook for another minute. Remove patties and add the rest of the ingredients into the same pan and cook on a medium heat until done. Pour the other ingredients over the fish and serve immediately.

6. ZUCCHINI NESTS WITH BACON, EGG & CHEESE

This delicious variant will surprise you as to how good it is. The zucchini becomes more like hash browns and the final product is tasty and fun to make while being fully Keto.

Ingredients:

- ✓ 1 zucchini, peeled & shredded into thin strips similar to spaghetti

- ✓ 4 eggs, whisked together with a dash of salt & pepper

- ✓ 6 strips of organic bacon (raw) cut into strips (thin)

- ✓ ½ cup grated Asiago cheese

- ✓ ¼ cup coconut oil

- ✓ 1 avocado peeled, diced into small cubes

- ✓ ¼ cup parmesan cheese

- ✓ 1 teaspoon basil

- ✓ 1 pinch of salt for each zucchini nest

- ✓ 1 teaspoon turmeric

- ✓

Directions:

Take the thin strips of zucchini and spin with a fork like you would do with spaghetti if you were about to eat it. Make small "nests" about 1 inch high.

Place the nests on a flat cookie sheet and drizzle coconut oil through the nest, dividing the ¼ cup of coconut oil among them.

Now add bacon and avocado to the nests. Sprinkle the remaining ingredients over the nests and finally pour the eggs over each nest. Cook in the oven for 20 minutes on 350 degrees.

7. MUSHROOMS & EGG SCRAMBLE WITH NOTES OF ORANGE

This Keto recipe was given to me by a lady in her 80s. She didn't know it was Keto, but I sure did. This is a flavorful and tasty new experience and will leave you happy and filled.

Ingredients:

- ✓ 4 eggs whisked with a dash of salt and pepper
- ✓ 6 slices of organic bacon, sliced in thirds
- ✓ 2 cups of organic white mushrooms, sliced
- ✓ ½ of a large orange, juiced
- ✓ ½ tablespoon fresh orange zest
- ✓ 1 tablespoon coconut oil
- ✓ ¼ cup heavy whipping cream

Directions:

Cook bacon until crisp, set aside. In a fry pan on a medium heat add mushrooms with scallions and coconut oil and cook for several minutes. Now add the egg mix and scramble.

Just as the eggs are almost done, add all remaining

ingredients. It is important that you follow this step for the right consistency and flavor.

Once the scramble is consistent, finish on a medium flame and set aside for a few minutes to let the ingredients set properly.

Variant:

Add salsa and remove the whipping cream.

8. SIMPLE EGGS WITH PORTOBELLO MUSHROOMS

Here we have a smaller version similar to the last recipe, which is easier to make. This makes a quick breakfast and still keeps you in the Keto zone:

Ingredients:

- ✓ 2 large eggs, cooked over easy in a teaspoon of coconut oil

- ✓ 1 Sweet & Sassy Keto Breakfast Pork Patties (see recipe 3)

- ✓ 2 large Portobello mushrooms diced

- ✓ ½ avocado diced

- ✓ 2 cups spinach leaves

- ✓ 1 tablespoon coconut oil

- ✓ ½ cup salsa, mild or to taste

Directions:

As mentioned earlier, now that you can make Keto sausage patties, we would explore using them in other recipes. If you prefer a variant, skip the patties and use 4 strips of organic bacon.

Crumble the Keto patties (or bacon substitute) on a plate over the spinach. Set aside.

Now cook the mushrooms in a small fry pan with the coconut oil. Cook for several minutes until tender. Add salt and pepper and add to the plate.

Finally cook the eggs and place on top of the ingredients on the plate and add salsa.

9. FETA PEPPERED GREEK EGGS & TOMATOES

Many people on the Keto lifestyle grow to live this flavor so much, it becomes a staple. You will love it too and once you try it you may never feel the same way about Greek eats (unless you already love it).

Ingredients:

- ✓ 4 eggs whisked together with a dash of salt

- ✓ 4-6 oz pre-cooked lamb (optional)

- ✓ 1 teaspoon organic black ground pepper

- ✓ ½ small white onion thoroughly diced

- ✓ ½ cup Feta cheese

- ✓ 1 tablespoon coconut oil

- ✓ ½ clove of garlic, minced

- ✓ ½ cup of cherry tomatoes

- ✓ 2 strips of organic bacon, cooked and crumbled

- ✓ 1 tablespoon of organic Greek salad dressing to taste

- ✓

<u>**Directions:**</u>

In a fry pan, add coconut oil and onion, clove of garlic and the pepper. Cook on a medium heat for about 2 minutes.

Now add the bacon and egg mix and scramble, folding the mix often.

Place cooked eggs on a plate and garnish with the Feta cheese and tomato.

To really get your "Greek" on, add the salad dressing. Also, some people like to add some lamb with their eggs as well.

10. ALMOND BREAKFAST MUFFINS

These muffins are not only delicious but portable, Keto approved and they make great snacks as well as a good meal for breakfast. Mix 'em together and do a quick bake for a dozen of these beauties:

Ingredients:

- ✓ 1¼ cups blanched almond flour

- ✓ ½ teaspoon Himalayan sea salt or plain sea salt

- ✓ ½ teaspoon baking soda

- ✓ 3 eggs

- ✓ ¼ cup almond slivers

- ✓ 2 tablespoons coconut oil

- ✓ 1 tablespoon coconut oil for greasing cupcake tray

- ✓ 1 tablespoon coconut flakes

- ✓ 6 strips organic bacon crumbled

- ✓ 1 cup grated parmesan cheese

- ✓ 2 teaspoons Stevia

- ✓ 1 teaspoon vanilla

Directions:

In a medium mixing bowl, pre-sift blanched almond flour until even consistency. Add eggs first and then vanilla; give about 30 strokes with a large spoon and add almond slivers, coconut oil, stevia and coconut flakes.

In a coconut oil greased cupcake pan, scoop about two tablespoons of batter and bake at 350 for about 15 minutes.

Garnish with crumbled bacon just as they come out of the oven.

11. POWER BERRY VANILLA KETO PANCAKES

Yes, you can have pancakes on the Keto lifestyle, if you make them like this. Once you add the berries, and top them with the whipping cream, you are golden.

Ingredients:

- ✓ 4 egg yolks
- ✓ 1 ½ cups of cottage cheese
- ✓ 1 tablespoon of unbleached flour
- ✓ 1 tablespoon almond flour
- ✓ 2 tablespoons of coconut oil
- ✓ 1 teaspoon vanilla extract
- ✓ 1 cup blackberries

Topping:

- ✓ ¼ cup raspberries
- ✓ 1 cup heavy whipping cream
- ✓ 1 teaspoon Stevia

Directions:

In a mixing bowl add all the ingredients and mix

with about 20 strokes. Do not over mix.

Cook on a hot skillet using coconut oil until it bubbles on the sides and flip. Cook until golden brown. Mix topping together and top.

12. KETO COCONUT PORRIDGE WITH SWEET CRÈME

Many of us still love a good bowl of porridge. Unfortunately, it can be high in carbs. Well, worry no more! Try this and enjoy that hearty flavor. Add fruit and a bit of heavy whipping cream with a touch of Stevia and you are golden!

Ingredients:

- ✓ 2 ½ tablespoons coconut flour, sifted if possible
- ✓ 2 tablespoons flax meal or psyllium husks
- ✓ ¾ cup water
- ✓ 1 egg whisked until even consistency
- ✓ 2 teaspoons natural butter (preferred) or 2 tablespoons coconut oil
- ✓ 1 tablespoon heavy cream or coconut milk
- ✓ 1 teaspoon Stevia
- ✓ ¼ cup favorite berries (suggest blueberries)

Directions:

In a medium saucepan add the coconut flour, flax meal (or psyllium husks) and water. Heat on a low heat until it begins to simmer.

Now add butter (or coconut oil) and slowly whisk in the egg over about a minute (this will incorporate the egg without scrambling it).

Finally add Stevia to heavy whipping cream and the fruit of your choice. Raspberries are also a good variant so try this.

Stevia is a good natural sweetener that also has health properties. Do not use any other sweetener.

13. MUSHROOM OMELET WITH PORK SAUSAGE & SPICES

One of the best, tasty omelets is a medley of spices with Keto sausage. You have to try this as it took quite some time and experimentation to get the flavors just right.

Ingredients:

- ✓ 3 eggs whisked with a dash of salt and pepper
- ✓ 2 tablespoons of coconut oil
- ✓ ¼ cup shredded cheddar cheese
- ✓ ½ small white onion diced thoroughly
- ✓ 1 Keto pork sausage, (recipe 3 in this guide) crumbled
- ✓ 1 cup diced mushrooms
- ✓ ½ clove of garlic minced
- ✓ 1 teaspoon rosemary
- ✓ 1 teaspoon basil
- ✓ 1 teaspoon allspice
- ✓ 1 teaspoon sage

Directions:

This recipe is simple. In a fry pan add 1 tablespoon of coconut oil, the garlic, the mushrooms and the allspice. Cook on medium heat for about 3 minutes and set aside.

Next add the crumbled keto pork sausage to the fry pan and cook for about 1 minute on a medium heat. Now add the eggs, mushrooms and the rosemary, basil and sage.

Cook until firm, flip and finish using remaining coconut oil.

14. SEAFOOD OMELET

Believe it or not, having seafood for breakfast is a good way to get going in the morning. Not only will you be getting protein you need, but plenty of Omega 3s too, -- just what the doctor ordered.

Ingredients:

- ✓ ½ package (about 6 oz.) of pre-cooked seafood like shrimp or crab

- ✓ 2 tablespoons olive oil

- ✓ 3 eggs, whisked with a dash of salt and pepper

- ✓ ½ green pepper, diced

- ✓ 1 clove of garlic, minced

- ✓ 1 tablespoon natural butter

- ✓ ½ tablespoon flax seeds

- ✓ ½ tablespoon diced chives

- ✓ 3 strips of organic bacon, cooked & crumbled

- ✓ 3 tablespoons olive oil-based mayonnaise

Directions:

In a flat pan or skillet, heat bacon, cook and

crumble. Leave fat from bacon in pan and add the natural butter.

Now cook the eggs in the flat pan, flipping the omelet base on both sides. Remove to a plate ready to receive the other ingredients.

Now add seafood, garlic, green pepper and chives. Cook on a low heat for several minutes stirring frequently.

Add the finished seafood mix to a prep bowl and add mayonnaise, flax seeds and bacon. Mix for about 20 strokes with a large spoon.

Dish out mixture on omelet round and fold in half.

15. KETO CHEESE N' SAUSAGE BREAKFAST OMELET

This delicious omelet was revealed to me while traveling on Route 66. It was intended to be a Paleo breakfast, but when you add more healthy fats and some new spices, it is simply delicious.

Ingredients:

- ✓ 3 eggs whisked with a dash of salt and pepper

- ✓ 2 tablespoons of coconut oil

- ✓ 1 Keto pork sausage, (recipe 3 in this guide) crumbled

- ✓ 3 strips of bacon, cooked & crumbled organic plus the fat from cooking

- ✓ ¼ cup shredded cheddar cheese

- ✓ ¼ cup mozzarella cheese

- ✓ 2 tablespoons parmesan cheese

- ✓ 1 chive, diced

- ✓ 1 teaspoon allspice

- ✓ 1 teaspoon garlic powder

Directions:

Using one tablespoon of coconut oil, heat a medium omelet skillet and add egg mix cooking on a medium heat.

Flip omelet round and finish cooking and set on a plate.

Now add remaining ingredients into the same pan and cook on a low heat (important to use low heat) for about two minutes.

Add contents from the pan to the plate and fold in half and serve immediately.

16. KETO BACON & EGG SPINACH CUPCAKES

Bacon cupcakes? Think them as mini "bread" filled with Keto goodness. Not only are these tasty, but they are easy to bring with you for later meals or snacks on the fly.

Ingredients:

- ✓ 8 eggs whisked with a dash of salt and pepper
- ✓ 4 tablespoons of coconut oil
- ✓ 1 tablespoon olive oil
- ✓ 1 teaspoon baking powder
- ✓ 1 cup spinach leaves fresh, chopped
- ✓ ½ cup sharp cheddar cheese
- ✓ 12 strips of organic bacon, cooked and crumbled
- ✓ 1½ cups almond flour
- ✓ 1 tablespoon sun dried tomatoes, diced
- ✓ 1 clove of garlic minced
- ✓ 1 teaspoon Stevia

Directions:

Grease a cupcake cooking tray with coconut oil and set aside.

In a large mixing bowl combine all of the dry ingredients plus the bacon, spinach and tomato.

Mix thoroughly and add coconut oil, olive oil, cheese and garlic. Mix until incorporated fully and then start spooning about a tablespoon for each cupcake slot in the baking pan.

Cook at 350 for 15 minutes.

17. VERY BERRY COOL KETO CRAPES

If you love crepes but thought you couldn't have them on the Keto lifestyle, think again. Not only are these super tasty but are some the healthy crepes you can make. So, go ahead and splurge. Keto also means delicious food!

Ingredients:

- ✓ The Crepe batter – (use coconut oil to cook)

- ✓ ½ packet of cream cheese, organic if possible

- ✓ 3 eggs, whisked with a dash of just salt

- ✓ 2 tablespoons almond flower

- ✓ 1 teaspoon Stevia

- ✓ 1 teaspoon cinnamon

- ✓ 1 teaspoon baking soda

- ✓ ½ teaspoon vanilla extract

Filling – (mix in a separate bowl and add to crepes, rolling)

- ✓ ½ package of cream cheese (the other half)

- ✓ ¼ cup blackberries, organic

- ✓ ¼ cup raspberries, organic

✓ dash of salt

✓ ½ teaspoon vanilla extract

<u>Directions:</u>

Mix all ingredients for the crepes first. Stir for about 30 beats until it runs like maple syrup. Heat the skillet until a drop of water dances on the surface. Cook about a tablespoon of batter quickly on a medium heat, flipping as soon as it bubbles on the edges. Cook until slightly brown and rubbery.

Now add 2 tablespoons of filling and roll like open burritos and serve.

18. EGG BAKE WITH BERRIES

Egg bakes are simple. Just add the ingredients into a skillet and bake, -- perfect for a quick breakfast. Some people even cook these ahead of time or prepare the bake and pop it in the oven when they are ready.

Ingredients:

- ✓ 6 eggs partially whisked (10 strokes) with a dash of salt and pepper

- ✓ 2 tablespoons natural butter

- ✓ 1 tablespoon coconut oil

- ✓ 3 tablespoons coconut flower

- ✓ ½ teaspoon vanilla extract

- ✓ 1 teaspoon orange zest

- ✓ 1 sprig (small) parsley minced

- ✓ ½ cup berries of your choice

- ✓ 1 teaspoon rosemary, minced

- ✓ ½ teaspoon Stevia (add last as instructed)

Directions:

Preheat oven to 350 degrees.

In a small crock / huge ramekin or Pyrex baking dish with a lid, place butter first and then ½ of the egg mix.

Partially cook eggs first for several minutes and add a dash of salt and pepper again.

Remove from oven for just a moment and add everything else.

Gently stir the bake and add berries last. Sprinkle dash of Stevia last and add the remaining eggs and stir. Cook for 10 minutes and serve.

19. POACHED EGGS WITH KETO SAUCE ON SPINACH

Even though this recipe sounds hard to make, it really isn't. This is a real treat, and if you are having company for breakfast, I would serve this.

Ingredients:

- ✓ 1 hot water egg poacher (or hand poach)

- ✓ 2 eggs, used in the poacher for poaching

- ✓ 1 cup spinach leaves, fresh and cut into a bed of strips

- ✓ 2 slices of bacon, organic pre-cooked

- ✓ 2 slices of fat ham (cut from a shank if possible) precooked.

"Hollandaise" Keto Sauce:

- ✓ 2 egg yolks

- ✓ ½ tsp Dijon mustard

- ✓ 2 tablespoons of fresh squeezed lemon juice

- ✓ ¼ cup extra virgin olive oil

- ✓ 1 tablespoon hot water as needed to thin out the mix

✓ 1 tablespoon Sriracha sauce

✓ dash salt & pepper to taste

Directions:

Poach eggs as directed and place on a plate over the bed of spinach and on top of the ham.

In a small saucepan, mix all of the sauce over a LOW heat and constantly and gently whisk for about 5 minutes, with less heat and time as the sauce thickens. Pour the mix over the eggs and serve immediately.

20. KETO CEREAL AND / OR KETO BREAKFAST BARS

Wow! Now you can have that super crunchy and sweet, satisfying cereal or breakfast bar in the morning or anytime. This recipe can be made and used anytime you crave a sweet & crunchy breakfast treat; only you will know it is low in carbs and almost zero sugar and perfectly nutritious.

Ingredients:

- ✓ ½ cup slivered almonds
- ✓ ¼ cup walnuts
- ✓ 2 tablespoons of coconut oil
- ✓ 1 tablespoon of coconut flakes
- ✓ 2 tablespoons of chia seeds
- ✓ 1 tablespoon of flax seeds
- ✓ 1 teaspoon Stevia
- ✓ 1 tablespoon of coconut flour
- ✓ 1 cup almond milk

Directions:

Mix all of the nuts / seeds with the coconut oil and add coconut flour. Mix completely and then add the remaining ingredients except the almond milk, which you will add when ready to eat as cereal.

Alternate Breakfast Bar without the almond milk:

- ✓ 1 teaspoon of cinnamon to the above recipe.

At this point you can also add the ingredients to a small baking pan and bake for 30 minutes on 350. Makes about 3 breakfast bars.

21. FLAXSEED, CINNAMON & EGG FIBER BREAKFAST MUFFINS

As you may know, flaxseed is very healthy for you. Muffins with flaxseed and other natural additives can heal your body and they actually taste great. Try this recipe and you will also be more regular (if you know what I mean).

Ingredients:

- ✓ 3 eggs, whisked together with a dash of salt
- ✓ 2 tablespoons psyllium husks
- ✓ ¼ cup coconut or almond flour
- ✓ 2 tablespoons of coconut oil
- ✓ 1 cup flaxseeds ground
- ✓ 2 teaspoons Stevia
- ✓ ½ teaspoon baking powder
- ✓ 1 teaspoon cinnamon
- ✓ 1 teaspoon vanilla extract
- ✓ 2 teaspoons almond milk

Directions:

In a medium mixing bowl, place all dry ingredients and dry mix until fully incorporated (well mixed).

Now add all the wet ingredients and beat with a wooden spoon for about 30 strokes.

Preheat oven to 350 degrees. Grease a cupcake baking tin and spoon about 1 well-rounded tablespoon into the cupcake wells.

Cook for 15 minutes or until a toothpick comes out clean from the center of one of the cupcakes.

22. KETO ENGLISH MUFFINS FOR BREAKFAST OR ANYTIME

Never thought you could have English muffins again? Think again. These simple 1-minute English muffins taste almost like the real McCoy. These are simple to make and once toasted, crisp on the outside and soft on the inside.

Ingredients:

- ✓ 1 tablespoon of unsalted natural butter
- ✓ 2 tablespoons of almond butter
- ✓ 2 tablespoons of almond or coconut flour
- ✓ ½ teaspoon baking powder
- ✓ 1 tablespoon unsweetened almond milk
- ✓ 1 egg with a dash of salt
- ✓ 1 tablespoon almond milk

Directions:

In a medium mixing bowl, microwave the first two ingredients (natural butter & almond butter) for 30 seconds on high. Stir until it runs smooth. Set aside.

In another mixing bowl, add the flour, baking flour and a dash of salt. Next add the almond milk and the egg and whisk thoroughly. Take the first bowl and add it to the second. Fully incorporate the two together. The final consistency should run like warm syrup.

Split the mix into two medium English muffin size ramekins (small, round microwave safe mini bowls) and microwave each for one minute on high until spongy. You can now remove the "hockey puck" and cut in half and toast just like English muffins / bread!23. Bacon Egg, Cheese & Coconut Crusted Ham, English Muffins

It is a mouthful to say but once you taste it, you will love this delicious breakfast sandwich. The crusted ham makes sure you get the additional high-quality fats.

Ingredients:

- ✓ 1 Keto English muffin, toasted (see recipe 22)

- ✓ 2 tablespoons of coconut oil

- ✓ 1 tablespoon coconut flakes, unsweetened

- ✓ ¼ cup coconut flakes unsweetened

- ✓ 1 slice of ham, lightly salted and diced

- ✓ 1 egg barely scrambled

✓ 1 thin slice sharp cheddar

✓ 2 strips of cooked bacon, organic

Directions:

Place one half of the English muffin on a plate and add the cheddar slice. Microwave for ten seconds and then set aside.

Now add one tablespoon of coconut oil to a small fry pan and partially scramble egg leaving it in mostly intact (do not over scramble but cook it thoroughly so it won't fall apart on the sandwich).

In the same fry pan, place 1 tablespoon of coconut oil, the coconut flakes and the slice of ham. Cook both sides, stirring until the oil absorbs most of the coconut oil. Place bacon on top of the cheese, followed by the coconut encrusted ham and the egg. Serve immediately.

24. PERFECT SCRAMBLED EGGS & SAUSAGE WITH ENGLISH MUFFIN

This classic breakfast has been made perfect by Keto recipes that combine other flavorful scrambles. You will love this combination so much it just might become your favorite.

Ingredients:

- ✓ 1 Keto sausage (recipe 3)

- ✓ 1 Keto English muffin toasted & buttered (see recipe 22)

- ✓ 1 tablespoon coconut oil

- ✓ 5 eggs, whisked with a dash of salt and pepper

- ✓ 2 tablespoons of natural, salt free butter

- ✓ 2 tablespoons of sour cream

- ✓ 1 tablespoon diced scallions

- ✓ 4 strips organic bacon

- ✓ ½ teaspoon garlic powder

- ✓ ½ teaspoon onion powder

- ✓ 1 dash paprika

- ✓ 1 dash Stevia

Directions:

Add coconut oil to a medium skillet and cook bacon in the oil. Do NOT drain fat and remove bacon. Now add eggs and start cooking for about 1 minute on a medium heat.

Next add all remaining ingredients, including the bacon (crumbled), except the sausage, which you need to heat up last and put on the English muffin.

Fold eggs / remaining ingredients continuously, until the food begins to thicken. Add on top of English muffin and sausage.

25. MINI KETO QUICHES WITH SUN DRIED TOMATO & BASIL

This fun recipe can yield several of these quiches to heat and eat anytime. The flavor will surprise you because eating Keto need not be bland.

Ingredients:

- ✓ 12 eggs, whisked together with 1 teaspoon pepper & ½ teaspoon salt

- ✓ ¼ cup sun dried and crumbled tomatoes, sun dried or dehydrated

- ✓ ¼ teaspoon of cayenne pepper

- ✓ 1 teaspoon tomato paste

- ✓ 1 teaspoon basil

- ✓ ½ cup mozzarella

- ✓ 1 diced jalapeño (optional but adds zing)

- ✓ ½ teaspoon Stevia

- ✓ 1 teaspoon olive oil

- ✓ 1 tablespoon coconut oil

- ✓ 5 strips of bacon cooked & crumbled (add bacon fat as well)

Directions:

Add all ingredients to a mixing bowl and beat for about 30 strokes.

Preheat oven to 350.

Into 2-3 large ramekins or 1 flat pie tin, pour ingredients and bake for for 25 minutes. Allow quiche to cool for 30 minutes or pop in the freezer for 15 minutes.

One variant is to also add ¼ cup of sharp cheddar and the bacon crumbles on the top of the quiche.

26. HAM EGG & 2 CHEESE COCONUT FRIED ROLLUPS

While this might sound fattening, on the Keto you need lots of healthy fats. Using coconut oil to fry these beauties (pan fried) makes them crispy, delicious and even nutritious. So, if you are looking for a real treat, give this a try.

Ingredients:

- ✓ 6 flour torts, (burrito wraps large) low carb or made from coconut flour

- ✓ 12 slices ham, preferably from the shank but slices will do

- ✓ 12 eggs whisked with a dash of salt and pepper

- ✓ 1 tablespoon of coconut oil for cooking eggs

- ✓ 3 cups of baby spinach leaves (1/2 cup per tort)

- ✓ 12 strips of bacon, organic cooked (2 each tort)

- ✓ ½ cup sour cream

- ✓ 3 scallions diced

- ✓ 3 tomatoes, organic diced

- ✓ 3 cups sharp cheddar (1/2 cup each tort)

- ✓ 3 cups Monterey jack cheese (1/2 cup each tort)

- ✓ Pinch of Stevia for topping on torts (each)

- ✓ ½ cup coconut oil for cooking

Directions:

Add a tablespoon of coconut oil in a medium to large skillet and then the eggs. Add the sour cream and more pepper (to taste) plus the scallions, cooking on a medium heat until scrambled. Set aside. Now cook bacon and drain grease in the egg mix. Crumble.

On a tort add everything else (divide ingredients as mentioned for each wrap) and roll tight into a burrito. In a large skillet add coconut oil and fry the burritos on high heat for several minutes on both side and set on paper towels. Garnish with Stevia and serve immediately.

27. CAULIFLOWER PEPPER HASH BROWNS

I know you miss hash browns on the Keto lifestyle, but these are almost as good if you follow the directions. They are also going to be healthy and tasty so you'll never miss out again.

Ingredients:

- ✓ 1 head of cauliflower, shredded with a cheese collider (make strips)
- ✓ 1 cup sharp cheddar
- ✓ 1 egg whisked with dash of pepper & salt
- ✓ ½ teaspoon of black pepper
- ✓ ½ teaspoon white pepper
- ✓ dash of cayenne pepper
- ✓ ¼ cup coconut oil for cooking

Directions:

In a medium mixing bowl, add all ingredients and stir gently until everything is incorporated.

Set aside.

In a medium to large skillet, add coconut oil and heat on high (be careful of heat).

Add 2 tablespoons of the cauliflower mix to a hot skillet and press flat like a pancake. Cook until golden brown on both sides.

You can also add tabasco sauce for a real zing or salsa once the cauliflower is cooked.

28. CLOUD BREAD FOR BREAKFAST / LUNCH / DINNER

Many of us grew up on bread. It is very satisfying to eat but has way too many carbs. Well NOT this bread! You only need three ingredients for this but you have to follow the directions carefully . . . so we put everything you need in the ingredients list for ease of understanding.

Ingredients:

- ✓ 3 eggs, separated whites from the yolks

- ✓ 2 medium mixing bowls: one for yolks, the other for the whites

- ✓ 1 cookie tray lined with wax paper

- ✓ 3 tablespoons of cream cheese, at room temperature

- ✓ 1 teaspoon of baking powder

Directions:

Preheat oven to 350 and set up cookie tray with wax paper on it. In the bowl with the yolks (do this first) add the cream cheese and whip on medium high until incorporated completely. Using room temperature cream cheese is critical for this to work right.

Clean mixer beaters in cold water and refrigerate beaters until cold to the touch before going to the egg whites. In the bowl with the egg whites add the baking powder and whip on medium to high until the consistency of Meringue (like cool whip and will stand up on its own).

Carefully fold both bowls of ingredients together preserving as much air as possible. Now add a dollop of the mix on the wax paper the size of the cloud bread that you want. Cook for 10 minutes and then 1 minute on broil to brown the top.

29. CREAM CHEESE KETO PANCAKES WITH "WHIPPED CREAM" TOPPING

What could be better for breakfast than pancakes? Well give these a try and you won't believe just how good Keto pancakes can be.

Ingredients:

- ✓ 2 eggs whisked
- ✓ 3 tablespoons cream cheese
- ✓ ½ cup coconut flour
- ✓ 1 dash vanilla extract
- ✓ ½ teaspoon baking powder
- ✓ ½ teaspoon Stevia
- ✓ 1 tablespoon coconut oil
- ✓ ½ teaspoon cinnamon

Topping:

- ✓ ½ cup heavy whipping cream
- ✓ ½ teaspoon line juice
- ✓ ½ teaspoon Stevia
- ✓ ½ teaspoon vanilla extract

Directions:

Mix flour and baking powder first, then everything else for about 30 beats with a large wooden spoon. Do not over mix and leave reasonably thick. Heat skillet until a drop of water dances on it and add coconut oil. Add about a tablespoon of batter and cook until golden brown. In a mixing bowl add topping ingredients, blend on high until fluffy and serve on the pancakes.

30. SAUSAGE, EGG & HAM PATTY WITH BREAKFAST SANDWICH

Here is a great combination to round off our final breakfast recipe. Using recipes 3 & 28 will finish this one, recipe 30.

Ingredients:

- ✓ 1 Keto sausage patty (see recipe 3)

- ✓ 2 slices of cloud bread (see recipe 28)

- ✓ ¼ cup sharp cheddar

- ✓ 1 egg

- ✓ ½ tablespoon coconut oil

- ✓ ½ of a medium avocado sliced in wedges

- ✓ 1 slice of ham preferably from a ham shank

Directions:

Prepare the Keto sausage as directed in recipe 3. Prepare the cloud bread as in recipe 28.

Cook the single egg in a small fry pan using the coconut oil and cook on a medium heat. Cook the egg until it is over hard so it won't explode when you bite down in the sandwich.

Next add the cloud bread, the cheese on both

slices and microwave for about ten seconds to melt the cheese slightly.

Last add ham & avocado.

Variant: Use the Keto English muffin recipe 22 instead of cloud bread.

DELICIOUS AND EASY TO PREPARE KETO DINNERS

This section includes quick and easy dinners / brunches. The idea is to make sure recipes are made of simple ingredients, yet complex enough for real flavor.

We do not include "lunch" because any of the dishes here can be used for that purpose as well because of ease of preparation.

We will start with some great slow cooker meals as they can be put in a crockpot and cooked on low while you are at work or out of the house for a few hours.

We also include complete meals and we are targeting about 4 people. If you want recipes for two people, simply cut the ingredients in half.

If you need to prepare for about 6 people add an additional 1/3 of everything, simple and fast.

Now lunch/dinner can be an experience without all the fuss!

1. SLOW COOKER BEEF 'N BROCCOLI FOR FOUR

This classic dinner is simple and easy to make. Keto means more natural fats which help your body remain in the correct zone. This meal is great on a cold day and is hearty.

Ingredients:

- ✓ 2 pounds of stock beef cubed for slow cooking
- ✓ 3 cups of water with beef stock (2 cubes)
- ✓ 3 scallions diced
- ✓ 2 teaspoons of Stevia
- ✓ 1 teaspoon fresh ginger
- ✓ ½ teaspoon Himalayan salt and organic ground black pepper
- ✓ 2 tablespoons coconut oil
- ✓ 1 tablespoon olive oil
- ✓ 3 garlic cloves, minced
- ✓ 1 teaspoon sesame seeds
- ✓ 1 teaspoon flax seeds
- ✓ 2 diced bell peppers

- ✓ 2 cups fresh broccoli

- ✓ 1 carrot diced

- ✓ 1 small white onion diced

Directions:

The beautiful thing about slow cooker meals are that everything usually goes into the pot and you set it on low and cook for at least 4-8 hours depending on ingredients. (this recipe is best at 6 hours)

A taste variant is to flash fry the beef with a pinch of Stevia and 1 tablespoon natural butter for additional taste.

2. DOUBLE BEEF & VEGGIES SLOW COOKER STEW

Slow cooker meals are wonderful for those of us on the move. Now you can add more beef and other veggies because this makes for a heartier meal.

Ingredients:

- ✓ 3 pounds of stock beef cubed for slow cooking

- ✓ 2 cups of water with beef stock (2 cubes)

- ✓ 1 teaspoon fresh ginger

- ✓ ½ teaspoon Himalayan salt and organic ground black pepper

- ✓ 2 tablespoons coconut oil

- ✓ 1 tablespoon olive oil

- ✓ 3 garlic cloves, minced

- ✓ 2 diced bell peppers

- ✓ 2 cups diced cauliflower

- ✓ 2 carrots diced

- ✓ 1 small white onion diced

- ✓ ½ cup of snap peas (uncooked, fresh)

- ✓ 1 tablespoon Worcestershire sauce

<u>**Directions:**</u>

Add all ingredients into slow cooker and cook on low for 6-8 hours. This is a great meal if you have to go to work. If you want to spice it up add about 1 /2 tablespoon hot sauce.

Another variant is to flash fry with coconut oil, the cubes of beef with a teaspoon of Stevia and garlic (2 cloves crushed).

Finally, a dash of coconut flour as you finish the flash fry carries the flavor into the stew.

3. CHEDDAR TAQUITOS WITH CLASSIC TACO SAUCE

Almost everybody loves Mexican cuisine. These simple but delicious taco "rolls" can also be fried with coconut oil to add some crunch and if you serve on a bed of diced tomatoes and romaine lettuce, are out of this world when it comes to flavor.

Ingredients:

- ✓ 1 pound of hamburger, free range

- ✓ 1 taco seasoning packet - try to get Taco Bell™ version if possible

- ✓ 1 cup diced Roma tomatoes

- ✓ 1 avocado cubed

- ✓ 12 small low carb flour torts OR almond / coconut torts

- ✓ 2 cups Mexican cheese (mix / 4 cheeses)

- ✓ 1 cup sour cream

- ✓ 1 cup coconut oil for flash frying of wrapped torts

- ✓ 1 cup salsa, mild (or hot if you prefer)

- ✓ ½ cup mild taco sauce

Directions:

Cook hamburger (do NOT drain fat), and seasoning (packet) and set aside.

Assemble the torts by adding all ingredients so as to divide them among the small torts you have. Roll tight and make sure they are closed (like taquitos).

Heat skillet with coconut oil and fry until golden brown. Serve on a bed of diced tomatoes and romaine lettuce with dipping taco sauce.

4. KETO PIZZA ROLLS

These simple fried and seasoned "rolls" are a great option to commercially produced toxic pizza rolls often sold in your grocer's freezer.

Ingredients:

- ✓ 5 small low carb torts
- ✓ ½ cup coconut oil
- ✓ ½ cup pepperoni diced
- ✓ 2 cups mozzarella cheese
- ✓ ¼ cup of pizza seasoning
- ✓ ¼ cup white onion minced
- ✓ ½ cup diced green peppers
- ✓ 1 Keto sausage, crumbled (see recipe 3)
- ✓ ½ cup pizza sauce

Directions:

On each tort place an even amount of the ingredients like you would with a burrito. The measurement above should be evenly divided.

Wrap the torts tightly and set aside.

Heat a medium or large skillet with the coconut oil.

Heat for about 5 minutes on a medium flame and take 2 torts at a time and flash fry them, turning in the pan until they are golden brown.

Remove torts onto a stack of paper towels and lightly sprinkle with additional pizza seasoning while hot.

One variant is to add hot sauce or jalapenos . . . hot, hot!

5. KETO BROCCOLI CHEESY FRIED TORT ROLLS

Similar to the last recipe, this one will make a good plan for dinner and you will have delicious leftovers that can be taken with you on the fly.

Ingredients:

- ✓ 5 large torts, low carb

- ✓ 3 cloves crushed & minced garlic

- ✓ ¼ cup organic true olive oil

- ✓ ¼ cup coconut oil for frying

- ✓ 2 cups shredded mozzarella cheese shredded

- ✓ ½ cup shredded Monterey jack and / or sharp cheddar (mix both)

Broccoli steamed:

- ✓ 2 cups diced / steamed fresh broccoli heads

- ✓ 1 teaspoon lemon pepper

- ✓ 1 tablespoon natural butter

Directions:

First steam broccoli (or heat up on stove with ¼ cup of water) and mix in lemon pepper and butter.

Next add olive oil and both cheeses. Mix well and scoop out enough mix for each burrito, wrapping them tight.

Heat a skillet on medium heat with the coconut oil. Pan fry each burrito until golden brown and serve immediately.

6. CHICKEN & PORK EAR SUPER KETO BAKE WITH VEGGIES

This modified classic chicken bake gets its inspiration from Shake 'n' Bake™. Once you add the cooking oils and use them to bind everything together you will love it.

Ingredients:

- ✓ 2 pounds boneless chicken breasts split into long strips

- ✓ 2 clear plastic bags for shaking chicken with spices

- ✓ 3 cups mixed veggies

- ✓ ½ teaspoon garlic powder

- ✓ ½ teaspoon onion powder

- ✓ ½ cup parmesan cheese

- ✓ ½ tablespoon Italian seasoning

- ✓ ½ teaspoon chicken bouillon (dry)

- ✓ ½ teaspoon chili pepper

- ✓ 2 cups crushed pigs ears

- ✓ 2 eggs whisked with a pinch of salt and pepper

✓ ½ cup coconut oil

✓ ¼ cup olive oil

Directions:

In a medium mixing bowl add all of the dry ingredients and incorporate everything together. Place dry ingredients in a bag.

Place veggies mixed with the oils on the bottom of a pyrex glass baking dish or lasagna pan.

Dip chicken on egg wash and then place in bag with dry ingredients and shake. Place chicken on a bed of the veggies and bake for 30 minutes, flipping chicken in about 15 minutes.

7. KETO WHIPPED "POTATOES"

Heavy carbs are a 'no – no' on the Keto lifestyle. Many of us crave potatoes and there is only one way to deal with this craving. . . Keto potatoes to the rescue!

Ingredients:

- ✓ 1 large or 2 medium cauliflower heads, steamed & crumbled

- ✓ ½ tablespoon potato flakes

- ✓ ½ cup whole milk

- ✓ 3 tablespoons natural butter

- ✓ ½ cup heavy cream

- ✓ 1 tablespoon coconut oil

- ✓ ½ teaspoon salt

- ✓ ½ teaspoon garlic salt

- ✓ ¼ teaspoon cracked or white pepper

- ✓ ¼ cup parmesan cheese

Directions:

In a medium mixing bowl add potato flakes and milk and one tablespoon of butter and 1 tablespoon coconut oil. Whip on medium speed for

30 seconds with a hand mixer.

Next add the cauliflower, salt, pepper and remaining 2 tablespoons of butter and whip for another 30 seconds on high.

Finally add heavy cream and parmesan cheese and whip on high for 2 minutes or until it reaches the the consistency of whipped potatoes.

You will still need to heat it up, so either microwave for 3 minutes on high or in a pot on the stove for several minutes on a medium flame stirring several times until everything is thick.

8. MEXICAN BEEF SKILLET

This simple recipe looks like it would be difficult but the directions are akin to a tossed salad. Try it and you will make this for dinner more than once.

<u>Ingredients:</u>

- ✓ 2 ripe avocados sliced into strips like potato wedges

- ✓ 1 teaspoon freshly squeezed lime juice

- ✓ 2 chives diced

- ✓ 1 small white onion diced

- ✓ 2 Roma or small cherub tomatoes diced

<u>The Beef:</u>

- ✓ 2 pounds of cubed stew beef

- ✓ 1 beef stock cube

- ✓ 1 tablespoon taco sauce

- ✓ ¼ cup olive oil

- ✓ ½ cup water

<u>Condiments:</u>

- ✓ 2 cups shredded lettuce

- ✓ ½ cup Mexican taco cheese

✓ 1 cup sour cream

<u>Directions:</u>

In a large fry pan on medium heat, cook all of the beef ingredients for about 5 minutes and remove from heat and place in a mixing bowl. Add remaining ingredients and gently stir together.

Preheat oven to 350 and place everything in an oven safe skillet and cook for 15 minutes. Serve immediately.

9. SPAGHETTI & MEAT SQUASH

Do you miss spaghetti? Here is a fun and delicious substitute that will make you think you are eating pasta when you are actually eating veggies.

Ingredients:

- ✓ 2 large Spaghetti squash
- ✓ 2 tablespoons coconut oil
- ✓ 1 pound of grass fed ground beef
- ✓ 1 cup Parmesan cheese
- ✓ 1 teaspoon chili powder
- ✓ 1 teaspoon Italian seasoning
- ✓ ½ teaspoon oregano
- ✓ 2 cloves of garlic, minced
- ✓ 3 cups pasta sauce
- ✓ ¼ cup coconut flour

Directions:

Cook spaghetti squash on 350 for an hour. Gut the squash in long strips (it tends to come out like this). Add to mixing bowl with coconut flour and coconut oil and gently fold with a spatula until thoroughly mixed.

Next cook beef with all the spices until brown. Do NOT drain fat and add spaghetti sauce.

Finally, place spaghetti squash on the plate first, add parmesan cheese (divide among servings).

Now add spaghetti sauce with meat on top and serve immediately.

You can add pepper flakes or chili spice for more zest.

10. LEBANESE CHICKEN THIGHS

Time for something really different with this classic Middle Eastern dish made to be 100% Keto compliant.

Ingredients:

- ✓ 4 chicken thighs with skins intact

- ✓ 2 cups of water

- ✓ 1 chicken bouillon cube

- ✓ ¼ cup garlic olive oil (or add two cloves of garlic to olive oil)

- ✓ 2 tablespoons natural butter

- ✓ 1 white onion quartered (do not dice)

- ✓ 2 carrots diced

- ✓ 2 celery stalks diced

- ✓ 2 small tomatoes cut in quarters

- ✓ 1 lemon juiced

- ✓ ¼ cup soy sauce

- ✓ 3 cups diced lettuce and field greens

Directions:

Preheat oven to 350. Mix all ingredients into a

small pyrex dish (with a lid) and mix all ingredients into a mixing bowl and pour over chicken.

Cover the bowl with the lid and cook for 30 minutes.

On a plate, put 2 thighs on about 2 cups of the greens and scoop a cup of the broth from the chicken and pour over it.

One variant is to add parmesan cheese over the greens.

Another variant is to add ½ a cup of olives.

Regardless, you will love the savory flavor so serve immediately.

11. CHICKEN KABOBS

Who doesn't love kabobs? They can be carried and eaten on a stick and each is a flavorful exploration of the world's best and delicious foods that also happen to be Keto.

Ingredients:

- ✓ 2 pounds of chicken, or lamb cut into kabob chunks

- ✓ 4 wooden skewers, cut veggies of choice to add to kabob.

Feta Marinade:

- ✓ 1 cup of Feta brine

- ✓ ½ cup olive oil

- ✓ ½ tablespoon lemon juice

- ✓ ½ teaspoon rosemary

- ✓ 3 cloves of garlic, minced

Italian Variant:

- ✓ ½ cup olive oil

- ✓ 1 lime, juiced

- ✓ ½ teaspoon chili powder

✓ ½ teaspoon onion powder

✓ 3 cloves of garlic, minced

<u>Directions:</u>

In a lasagna pan or rectangular Pyrex dish, place the ingredients for the marinade. Place chicken in dish and let stand for 4 hours at room temperature and for at least 12-24 hours in the refrigerator. When ready, grill for 5 minutes on each side on an outside grill. Make sure internal temperature of chicken reaches 140 degrees.

12. ITALIAN "BREADED" PORK CUTLETS

Pork cutlets are a good meal especially if you like them "breaded." Why is breaded in quotes? Well look at the recipe and you will understand.

Ingredients:

- ✓ 6 pork cutlets lightly salted and peppered

- ✓ ½ cup Italian dressing & ½ cup water in medium bowl

- ✓ ½ cup grated parmesan cheese

- ✓ 2 eggs whisked in medium bowl

- ✓ 1 cup crushed pigs ears

- ✓ 1 dash Italian seasoning

- ✓ 1 sprig of parsley

- ✓ ½ cup coconut oil

Directions:

Soak cutlets for 4 hours in Italian dressing and water at room temperature.

Preheat oven to 350 degrees. Dip cutlets in egg wash and then dip in parmesan and crushed pigs ears with a dash of Italian dressing.

Now place in the Pyrex dish and cover with coconut oil. Bake for 20 minutes.

You can garnish with parsley by dicing and adding on top of cutlets just before they finish cooking. You can also add a dash of applesauce and a touch of cinnamon for more flavor.

13. KETO POT ROAST WITH BROWN GRAVY & MASHED "POTATOES"

Pot roast with gravy & mashed potatoes is a staple in America. People love this meal especially on cold days. It reminds us of fall and winter. Try it today and see!

Ingredients:

- ✓ 1 medium pot roast, with "dry rub" applied
- ✓ 2 cups beef broth
- ✓ ½ cup olive oil or garlic olive oil
- ✓ 1 serving of Keto whipped "potatoes" see recipe 7 (Keto Dinners)

Rub:

- ✓ ½ teaspoon thyme
- ✓ ½ teaspoon tsp celery salt
- ✓ 1 teaspoon basil
- ✓ 2 teaspoon dried dill weed
- ✓ 2 teaspoons garlic powder
- ✓ 1 tablespoon oregano

Gravy:

- ✓ 1 cup meat drippings

- ✓ 1 packet brown gravy mix

Preheat oven to 350 degrees. Mix the ingredients for the rub and apply to the pot roast and put in a pot roast pan with a lid.

Cook for one hour and use meat drippings to make gravy. Prepare "potatoes" according to recipe 7 and plate it up. Enjoy!

14. CHICKEN SOUP BONE BROTH

Bone broth is actually very healthy for you. Plus, it can be seasoned to taste great. The next time you need a pick me up, try this:

Ingredients:

- ✓ 1 whole chicken medium to large
- ✓ 10 cups of water
- ✓ ½ yellow onion minced
- ✓ 1 tablespoon onion powder
- ✓ 2 tablespoons minced garlic
- ✓ 1 tablespoon garlic salt
- ✓ 1 teaspoon dried thyme
- ✓ 2 cups diced celery
- ✓ 1 tablespoon apple cider vinegar
- ✓ ½ cup coconut oil
- ✓ 2 chicken bouillon cubes

Directions:

In large pot place thawed whole chicken and cover with water, about 10 cups, more or less as needed. Boil for 1 hour and remove from stove. SAVE

WATER and filter with a strainer.

Separate the meat and the bones. Pour water back in the same pot and add JUST the large bones. Boil for 20 more minutes. DO NOT micro STRAIN *except* for any bone fragments.

Add the broth to another pot with the chicken and all the ingredients plus 2 chicken bouillon cubes. Cook on a low heat for 15 minutes.

Serve just like chicken soup. This is very healthy, low carb and nutritious.

15. CHICKEN VEGGIE CASSEROLE

This classic dinner is a snap and will also leave you happy and healthier than most dinners. Try this wonderful and flavorful variant and you will love it.

Ingredients:

- ✓ 2 boneless chicken breasts

- ✓ 3 tbsp natural butter

- ✓ 1 small white onion minced

- ✓ ½ tablespoon minced garlic

- ✓ 1 cup chicken stock (or chicken soup bone broth recipe 14-Keto Dinners)

- ✓ 1 pinch of parsley or diced sprig

Ingredients for Casserole:

- ✓ 3 cups cauliflower

- ✓ 1 cup heavy cream

- ✓ 1 tsp lemon juice

- ✓ ½ cup mayonnaise

- ✓ 3 cups steamed, chopped broccoli

- ✓ 2 cups shredded cheddar cheese

Directions:

Place first set of ingredients in a skillet on the stove and cook for about 5 minutes, flipping chicken in about half the time. Set aside.

Preheat oven to 350 degrees and place all casserole ingredients first, then the chicken and the rest on top. Cook for 30 minutes and remove and serve immediately.

16. BEST KETO MEATBALLS ON PLANET EARTH?

Well maybe not The best, but darn close. Try these, but pay close attention to the recipe because if you do you will love these.

Ingredients:

- ✓ 1 lb. ground beef, lamb or pork made / processed like hamburger
- ✓ ½ cup grated parmesan cheese
- ✓ ½ cup olive oil
- ✓ ½ cup ground pigs ears
- ✓ ½ tablespoon barbecue seasoning
- ✓ ½ packet sloppy joe seasoning
- ✓ ½ teaspoon white cracked pepper
- ✓ ½ teaspoon Himalayan salt
- ✓ 1 tablespoon minced garlic
- ✓ ½ cup mozzarella cheese
- ✓ 1 teaspoon onion powder

Directions:

In a medium mixing bowl, place all ingredients and

incorporate until the consistency of what you might use for hamburger patties.

Preheat oven to 350 degrees.

On a long cookie sheet roll about 2 tablespoons of the meat & spice mix into balls, about the size of golf balls.

Place on sheet and cook for 15 minutes. You can also turn these into hamburgers by simply changing their shape.

17. BEST HOT / MILD SLOW COOKER CHICKEN WINGS

Many people love wings. The best part is slow cooker recipes, which can add spice to your day and make cooking a snap.

Ingredients:

- ✓ 1 bag of chicken wings, unprocessed

- ✓ ½ stick natural butter (3-4 tablespoons)

- ✓ 1/4 cup hot sauce of choice OR ½ tablespoon paprika (non-hot)

- ✓ 2 cloves of garlic, minced

- ✓ ½ a lime, fresh squeezed

If you like honey add these ingredients:

- ✓ ½ cup of natural local honey

- ✓ ½ a lemon, fresh squeezed

If you like Barbecue sauce add these ingredients:

- ✓ 1 tablespoon barbecue spice

- ✓ ½ tablespoon apple cider vinegar

Directions:

Add the chosen ingredients into a slow cooker and cook on low for 4 hours. Finish on high for 30 minutes and remove. Serve with celery & bleu cheese.

You can also add a side of Keto ranch dressing for flavor.

18. MEAT BACON TACOS

Many people love bacon, so why not make these delicious bacon tacos? Not only these are fun to eat but very flavorful.

Ingredients:

- ✓ 1 pound of hamburger cooked

- ✓ 1 taco seasoning packet OR ¼ cup taco sauce

- ✓ ¼ cup taco sauce for garnish on the tacos

- ✓ ¼ cup ranch dressing

- ✓ 2 cups shredded thinly sliced lettuce

- ✓ ½ cup diced tomatoes

- ✓ 20 strips of bacon

- ✓ 2 eggs whisked

Directions:

On a plastic microwave bacon dish, lay out 5 strips of bacon over the cooking mold to form a "taco shell" or upside down "U." Brush with egg wash and microwave until it forms a shell, about 4 minutes.

Cook hamburger meat and add taco seasoning or

taco sauce.

Now add all ingredients to build a taco. This includes dividing all ingredients up among the 4 tacos you will make.

If you do not want all the bacon, you can substitute small torts.

Another possibility is to create a taco bowl out of this by adding the lettuce and diced bacon with all the rest of the ingredients in a small bowl.

Finally add a dash of tabasco sauce for a kick.

19. PHILLY CHEESE STUFFED COCONUT COATED PEPPERS

This is a delicious way to enjoy Philly cheese steak and get all of the good fats. Staying Keto has never been easier.

Ingredients:

- ✓ 4 medium green bell peppers
- ✓ 4 tablespoons of natural butter
- ✓ ½ cup white onion chopped
- ✓ 1 teaspoon minced garlic
- ✓ 1-pound shaved Philly steak
- ✓ 3 tablespoons coconut oil
- ✓ 1 cup Monterey Jack cheese
- ✓ 1 cup mozzarella
- ✓ 1 tablespoon of Italian dressing
- ✓ 2 tablespoons of mayonnaise

Directions:

In a large skillet place the coconut oil, Italian dressing and pre-cook for about 5 minutes. Set aside.

Preheat oven to 350 degrees.

Now cut peppers in half and place in a cooking tray. Mix steak with remaining ingredients.

Add a dash of salt and pepper and bake for 15 minutes.

Add steak sauce for a variant.

20. LEMON SQUASH "PASTA" WITH LAMB OR STEAK

This veggie dish is filled with good fats and some solid meat too. Lemon pepper makes it all sync together.

Ingredients:

- ✓ 1 pound of lamb or steak cubed
- ✓ 3 yellow summer squash
- ✓ 1 tablespoon lemon pepper seasoning
- ✓ 2 tablespoons olive oil
- ✓ 1 tablespoon coconut oil
- ✓ 2 cloves of garlic minced
- ✓ ¼ cup parsley diced
- ✓ ½ lemon fresh squeezed or juiced

Directions:

Preheat oven to 350 degrees. Cut squash in half and cook for 45 minutes on a cookie sheet.

On the stove pre-cook the meat of choice for several minutes with all of the ingredients except the squash.

Now add the scooped-out squash to the skillet and fold for about 10 minutes until everything is mixed well.

You can add some salt, but I suggest you skip the pepper.

You can also serve on a bed of romaine and spinach leaves as this flavor is more enhanced by adding some uncooked greens.

An additional variant is to cook a bit more meat for a heartier dinner, -- like 2 pounds instead of one.

21. KETO MEATLOAF

A good meatloaf is a joy unto itself. Simply add all ingredients and cook in the oven. In 30 minutes you have a meal for the entire family.

Ingredients:

- ✓ 2 lbs fatty ground beef
- ✓ 2 eggs
- ✓ 1 tablespoon coconut oil
- ✓ 2 tablespoons olive oil
- ✓ 1 tablespoon tomato paste
- ✓ ½ white onion minced
- ✓ ½ teaspoon Himalayan salt
- ✓ 4 cloves garlic minced
- ✓ ½ teaspoon Dijon mustard
- ✓ ½ cup crushed pigs ears
- ✓ ¼ cup parmesan cheese
- ✓ 1 tablespoon Worcestershire sauce
- ✓ ½ cup mozzarella cheese
- ✓ 1 tablespoon barbecue sauce

✓ ¼ cup sesame seeds or flax seeds

<u>Directions:</u>

In a large mixing bowl leave meat out for 1 hour to warm it up for ease of handling. Preheat oven to 350 degrees. Place all remaining ingredients and mix by hand. On a cooking sheet form the meatloaf with your hands making it look like a loaf of bread.

Cook for 30 minutes and garnish the top with the barbecue sauce and the seeds. Cook for another 5 minutes and then cool for 15 minutes before serving.

22. TUSCAN KETO CHICKEN

Tuscan flavor is not just for taste, but a lifestyle based on Tuscany, Italy. Here food and culture meet in a climatic medley of culture. Try this chicken and be whisked away . . .

Ingredients:

- ✓ 2 pounds boneless skinless chicken breasts, thinly sliced
- ✓ ½ lime fresh squeezed
- ✓ /12 teaspoon chili powder
- ✓ 2 tablespoons olive oil
- ✓ 1 tablespoon sunflower oil OR coconut oil
- ✓ 1 cup heavy cream
- ✓ ½ cup chicken broth
- ✓ 2 cloves of garlic minced
- ✓ 2 teaspoons Italian seasoning
- ✓ ½ cup parmesan cheese
- ✓ 1 cup fresh spinach leaves
- ✓ ½ cup sun dried tomatoes

Directions:

In a medium mixing bowl, place the chicken and lime with the chili powder and the sunflower or coconut oil. Stir until well coated.

Preheat oven to 360 degrees.

In a Pyrex baking dish or lasagna pan, place chicken strips on the bottom with the remnants from the mixing bowl over the chicken.

In the same mixing bowl add the remaining ingredients (everything else) and mix for about 30 beats with a wooden spoon. Pour / scrape everything and cover the chicken. Bake for 15 minutes, turn the chicken and bake for another 15 minutes. Serve immediately.

23. KETO SHRIMP ALFREDO

If you love shrimp Alfredo and still want to live the Keto lifestyle, you have to try this recipe. Simply mix the ingredients together and bake.

Ingredients:

- ✓ 2 pounds raw peeled shrimp (buy from local farms not China)

- ✓ 2 tablespoons natural butter

- ✓ ½ white onion diced

- ✓ 1 small packet cream cheese at room temperature

- ✓ 1 cup heavy cream

- ✓ ¼ cup whole milk

- ✓ 2 cloves of garlic minced

- ✓ 1 teaspoon basil

- ✓ 1 teaspoon salt

- ✓ ½ cup shredded Parmesan cheese

- ✓ ¼ cup olives, diced

- ✓ ½ tablespoon olive oil

- ✓ 2 sun dried tomatoes diced

✓ 1 cup baby spinach, fresh

<u>Directions:</u>

In a large skillet, add the shrimp, butter, salt and garlic. Cook for about 3 minutes on a medium heat, stirring occasionally. Next add the remaining ingredients except for the spinach. Stir often, folding until all ingredients are incorporated and a nice and savory white Alfredo sauce appears. Cook for about 5 minutes or less. Do NOT overcook or you will burn the sauce.

When the consistency runs like thick maple syrup, it should be ready and since you pre-cooked the shrimp, the flavors will complement the final dish with the shrimp cooked correctly.

24. BACON EGGPLANT ALFREDO

Eggplant can be made quite tasty with bacon and Alfredo sauce. If you need a different dish, here is one that is sure to please even family and friends.

Ingredients:

- ✓ 1-pound bacon

- ✓ 2 pounds eggplant, pre-cooked and cubed

- ✓ 1 tablespoon coconut oil

- ✓ 1 tablespoon olive oil

- ✓ 1 cup heavy cream

- ✓ 2 tablespoons natural butter

- ✓ 2 cloves garlic minced

- ✓ 1 tablespoon white wine (optional but it helps the taste)

- ✓ 1 tablespoon lemon juice

- ✓ 1 cup shredded Parmesan cheese

Directions:

Preheat oven to 350.

Add all oils to the bottom of the cooking dish with the coconut oil and olive oil drizzled over the eggplant.

Next add all the remaining ingredients into a mixing bowl and stir for about a minute until a smooth consistency.

Pour the mixing bowl contents over the eggplant. Cook for 30 minutes; remove and let cool for about 15 minutes. You can serve immediately or reheat later. The taste actually improves over time . . .

25. ZUCCHINI & ALMOND PESTO

Pesto is a great way to experience foods that are well ground and easy to digest. You can eat it straight or on low carb wraps / chips. You can also add it to other meals as a sauce or flavor enhancer.

Ingredients:

- ✓ 2 medium Zucchinis cut into cubes
- ✓ 1 avocado, cut, peeled & cubed
- ✓ ¼ cup walnuts
- ✓ ¼ cup fresh basil leaves
- ✓ ¼ cup almond slices
- ✓ 2 cloves garlic peeled
- ✓ ½ peeled lemon OR juiced
- ✓ ¼ cup grated Parmesan cheese
- ✓ 1 tablespoon olive oil
- ✓ ½ tablespoon Italian seasoning
- ✓ 1 pinch of Salt and pepper

Directions:

This recipe is easy to make. Simply place all of the ingredients in a food processor and grind until you have a smooth paste, about 30-45 seconds.

The pesto can be eaten cold like a dip.

You can add the pesto to other recipes for flavor and food enhancement. For example, baked chicken with the pesto on top.

I also suggest trying this pesto with Keto bread or low carb tort chips. Finally, you can add the pesto to wraps with meat like lamb or chicken for a quick meal.

26. MACHO NACHOS WITH STEAK & CHEESES

Nachos? Yes, you can have nachos if you use this recipe. Here's how to make your own like this.

Ingredients:

- ✓ 1-pound beef round tip steak
- ✓ 2 tablespoons natural butter
- ✓ ½ white onions minced
- ✓ 1 teaspoon chili powder

The "chips:"

- ✓ 2 medium torts
- ✓ 2 tablespoons of coconut oil
- ✓ ½ teaspoon turmeric

The Nacho Toppings:

- ✓ 1-pound cauliflower cooked & shredded
- ✓ ½ cup shredded cheddar cheese
- ✓ ½ cup shredded Monterey jack
- ✓ ½ cup sour cream
- ✓ ½ mashed avocado

✓ 2 tablespoons coconut oil

Directions:

In a large skillet, add the chips ingredients and cook until they begin to harden like regular chips, about 3 minutes on high flame. Remove.

Now add main steak ingredients and cook for several minutes on a high flame, mixing often and then remove. Repeat the process for macho toppings and assemble everything together like classic nachos. Enjoy!

27. CHICKEN SKILLET WITH HONEY & WALNUTS

This recipe is actually quite easy to make. Finally, here is a fantastic Keto recipe that is skillet based and sweet. With healthy fats and real honey, the flavor makes all the difference to your Keto lifestyle.

Ingredients:

- ✓ 2 chicken breasts cut into long strips
- ✓ 2 tablespoons of coconut oil
- ✓ 1 green pepper diced
- ✓ 1 tablespoon local honey
- ✓ ½ cup walnuts
- ✓ ½ teaspoon paprika
- ✓ 2 scallions diced

Salad:

- ✓ 2 cups thin chopped romaine
- ✓ 1 tablespoon ranch
- ✓ 1 tablespoon salad oil
- ✓ ½ tablespoon white vinegar or vinaigrette

- ✓ ½ tablespoon walnuts

- ✓ ½ tablespoon flax seeds

- ✓ 2-5 cherry tomatoes

Directions:

In a medium skillet, place all of the first set of ingredients and cook on a medium heat for about 5 minutes stirring occasionally. Plate up salad and add chicken and enjoy!

28. SWEET N' SOUR KETO MEATBALLS

These meatballs will add some sweet and sassy taste to any dinner table. Only you will know they are for your new Keto lifestyle, so cook them up and enjoy.

Ingredients:

The meatballs

- ✓ 1-pound ground beef
- ✓ 1 egg, whisked in a cup with a dash of salt and pepper
- ✓ ½ white onion minced
- ✓ ¼ cup Parmesan cheese
- ✓ ½ teaspoon garlic powder
- ✓ 1 teaspoon Worcestershire sauce

For the sauce

- ✓ 1 ½ cups water
- ✓ ¼ cup apple cider vinegar
- ✓ 3 tablespoons soy sauce
- ✓ ½ cup sugar free ketchup
- ✓ ½ teaspoon Stevia

Directions:

Let meat stand out of the refrigerator for about 1 hour to warm it up for ease of handling. Preheat oven to 350 degrees. In a mixing bowl add all of the meatball ingredients and mix with your hand. Form into golf ball sizes and place on cookie sheet.

For the sauce: simply mix it all together and whisk it for about 30 strokes. In a small saucepan, heat sauce for about 5 minutes on low heat. Pour over meatballs and serve when done.

29. KETO GYROS WITH RANCH & FETA CHEESE

Gyros can be a great dinner or a quick lunch too. They have delicious flavor and with the right combination of herbs, you too will be having them more and more.

Ingredients:

Gyro Meat

- ✓ 1-pound ground lamb
- ✓ 1 cup pork rinds or pigs ears
- ✓ 2 tablespoons coconut oil
- ✓ 1 cup feta cheese
- ✓ Himalayan salt & pepper to taste
- ✓ 1 tablespoon oregano
- ✓ 3 cloves garlic minced

Gyro Sauce and torts

- ✓ ½ cup low carb ranch
- ✓ 1 tablespoon coconut oil
- ✓ 1 tablespoon white vinegar
- ✓ 2 tablespoons olive oil

- ✓ ½ cup diced cucumbers, 4-6 flour torts, low carb or coconut

- ✓ 2 cups thin sliced in strips, romaine lettuce

Directions:

Use low carb wraps or coconut flour wraps. In a mixing bowl combine all of the gyro meat ingredients and hand mix thoroughly. Make into flat patties and cook in a skillet like hamburgers.

Combine all sauce ingredients and mix. Assemble gyros with cubed meat and pour sauce and add romaine lettuce. Enjoy!

30. ITALIAN SAUSAGE SKILLET BAKE WITH SALSA

This simple skillet meal is a snap to make and it is also a great dinner meal to make when time is short.

Ingredients:

- ✓ 4 Italian sausages diced OR Keto sausages (see recipe 3 in breakfast)

- ✓ 3 tablespoons Dijon mustard

- ✓ 2 garlic cloves minced

- ✓ 2 tablespoons coconut oil

Remaining Ingredients

- ✓ ½ cup heavy whipping cream

- ✓ ½ cup tomato sauce

- ✓ ½ cup water

- ✓ Dash Himalayan salt and white pepper

- ✓ 1 cup fresh spinach leaves

- ✓ ½ cup grated Parmesan cheese

- ✓ 1 teaspoon parsley flakes

- ✓ 1 cup shredded sharp cheese

✓   1 cup mild (or hot) salsa

Directions:

In a medium skillet: add sausages, mustard, garlic and coconut oil. Cook on a medium heat for several minutes then add the water and tomato paste.

Next add all remaining ingredients except the whipping cream. Cook for another few minutes on a medium flame and finally add the whipping cream and fold for about 1 minute. If you like it hot, add a dash of tabasco sauce. Serve immediately.

31. SKILLET CHICKEN WITH TASTY GREENS & CHEDDAR SAUCE

This final recipe is also a skillet meal and is a great way to substitute from mac n' cheese. The chicken makes the dish really work well.

Ingredients:

- ✓ 1-pound boneless chicken breasts cut into strips
- ✓ 2 tablespoons coconut oil
- ✓ 1 tablespoon Italian dressing

The Veggies & Spices

- ✓ 1 cup chicken stock
- ✓ 1 cup heavy cream
- ✓ 2 cups dark leafy baby spinach leaves
- ✓ 1 green pepper, diced
- ✓ 1 tablespoon diced chives
- ✓ 1 tablespoon olive oil
- ✓ 2 tablespoons coconut flour
- ✓ ½ teaspoon white pepper
- ✓ Dash Himalayan salt

<u>**Directions:**</u>

In a medium skillet, add the first set of ingredients (chicken) and cook for about 5 minutes on a medium flame. Set aside for a moment.

In a medium mixing bowl, add all remaining ingredients. Stir for a minute and then empty bowl into the skillet.

Cook for another 3 minutes on a medium heat mixing occasionally. Serve immediately.

KETO SNACKS BONUS SECTION

Snack yourself to health? Yes!

These snacks are great for life on the fly. Now you can pass temptation when you make these snack foods and take them with you.

Not only are these snacks are designed to be tasty, but finally you will have real choices to keep and maintain your Keto Lifestyle.

We also incorporated "superfoods" as part of these snacks so that the nutrition and healthiness is there. Never skip a meal again and use foods like this to maintain your Keto lifestyle.

1. KETO VANILLA OR CHOCOLATE RICH & CREAMY SHAKE

This is a simple way to have a meal replacement and enjoy either a chocolate or vanilla treat.

Ingredients:

- ✓ 2 scoops high quality chocolate or vanilla ice cream
- ✓ 1 tablespoon cocoa or vanilla powder
- ✓ 2 tablespoons coconut oil
- ✓ 1 tablespoon unsweetened chocolate or vanilla shavings
- ✓ 1 tablespoon of heavy cream
- ✓ 1 tablespoon coconut shavings
- ✓ ½ cup blueberries or raspberries

Directions:

Place all ingredients into a blender and blend until rich and creamy.

Variants:

Some people add two raw eggs and blend as well. You can also add liquid supplements to your morning shake such as vitamins.

If you want a tang to your shakes, add the juice of an orange and you have what is essentially an orange Julius™ but this will spike sugar.

I suggest using lime as this adds alkaline properties as well as vitamin C without the sugar. If you love orange use orange spice or orange zest and Stevia as a reasonable substitute.

Finally, lemon and lime are great additives with Stevia as well.

2. PORK RINDS MIX WITH NUTS

This simple snack includes superfoods (nuts) if you follow this easy mix. This is also good trail mix and can help keep you going throughout the day:

Ingredients:

- ✓ 1 cup pork rinds
- ✓ ½ cup dried fruit of choice (low glycemic)
- ✓ ½ cup almonds
- ✓ ½ cup almond slivers
- ✓ ½ cup sunflower seeds
- ✓ ½ cup chia seeds
- ✓ ½ cup flaxseeds
- ✓ ½ cup pumpkin seeds

Directions:

Thoroughly mix all ingredients in a medium mixing bowl and add to zip lock bags.

The snack is perfect for on the fly because it does not need refrigeration and will help you curb hunger and temptation.

Do NOT buy seeds that are processed with salt or

sugar and always favor seeds that have their skins intact wherever possible.

Other variants include adding coconut oil and baking the mix into bars that can then be eaten like a snack bar:

To Make A Snack Bar: add two tablespoons of coconut oil, 1 egg and1/2 tablespoon coconut flour. Mix, place in a small pan and cook at 350 for 15 minutes. Cut and refrigerate and serve as snack bar.

3. DARK CHOCOLATE & CRUNCHY SEED BAR

If you liked the last recipe, you are going to love this one. Here we make a mix that we bake and cut into delicious and sweet tasting chocolate. Not only is this extremely healthy, but there is no actual sugar and tons of protein.

Ingredients:

- ✓ ½ cup dark chocolate or similar unsweetened cocoa

- ✓ 1 egg, whisked with a pinch of Himalayan salt

- ✓ 1 teaspoon Stevia

- ✓ 2 tablespoons of natural butter

- ✓ 2 tablespoons of coconut oil

- ✓ 2 tablespoons coconut oil to grease a pan

- ✓ ½ cup coconut flour

- ✓ ½ cup dried fruit of choice (low glycemic)

- ✓ ½ cup almonds

- ✓ ½ cup almond slivers

- ✓ ½ cup sunflower seeds

- ✓ ½ cup chia seeds

- ✓ ½ cup flaxseeds

- ✓ ½ cup pumpkin seeds

Directions:

Place all ingredients in a medium mixing bowl and hand mix with a wooden spoon about 30 beats.

Preheat oven to 350 degrees. In a coconut greased pan, add the mix and bake for 15 minutes. Let cool for 1 hour and then cut into bars. Try these as meal replacements or for snacks.

4. DARK CHOCOLATE "PUDDING" A LA AVOCADO

Avocados make excellent pudding and when seasoned carefully they are almost indistinguishable from real carb laden puddings. Avocados are an excellent source of healthy fats and there is no baking involved.

Ingredients:

- ✓ 1 large avocado peeled and cubed
- ✓ ½ cup dark baking chocolate, unsweetened
- ✓ ½ tablespoon cocoa
- ✓ 1 teaspoon Stevia
- ✓ ½ teaspoon vanilla extract
- ✓ 1 tablespoon heavy cream
- ✓ 1 dash cinnamon
- ✓ 1 dash salt
- ✓ 1 dash nutmeg

Directions:

In a medium mixing bowl, mash the avocado and then mix all the remaining ingredients together, first with a wooden spoon and then finish with a hand mixer. You can serve immediately.

Whipped topping:

- ✓ 1 cup heavy whipping cream

- ✓ 1 teaspoon vanilla

- ✓ 1 teaspoon Stevia

Mix on high until it's whipped cream consistency. Add to pudding.

5. PEANUT BUTTER & CHOCOLATE BARS WITH ALMONDS

Inspired by several popular candy bars, here is a healthy variant you can easily make, mix and bake. Once done serve and you won't believe these are sugar free and almost carb free.

Ingredients:

- ✓ ½ cup organic peanut butter
- ✓ ½ cup baking chocolate unsweetened
- ✓ 1 tablespoon cocoa
- ✓ 1 teaspoon vanilla extract
- ✓ 1 teaspoon Stevia
- ✓ 1 egg
- ✓ ½ cup coconut flour
- ✓ 2 tablespoons natural butter
- ✓ 1 tablespoon coconut oil
- ✓ 2 tablespoons coconut oil to grease the pan
- ✓ ½ cup almonds

Directions:

In a medium mixing bowl, add all ingredients and

beat with a spoon until all ingredients look reasonably incorporated.

If necessary add a few pinches more of coconut flour until a thick consistency that will still run like pancake batter.

Preheat oven to 350 and in a greased small lasagna pan or pyrex dish, cook for 15 minutes.

6. KALE CHIPS WITH BARBECUE SEASONING

Making kale chips is easy and just requires a few minutes. You will be surprised at how good these are and with different seasoning you can change the flavor easily.

Ingredients:

- ✓ 1 bunch kale
- ✓ 2 tablespoons olive oil
- ✓ 2 tablespoon Parmesan cheese
- ✓ 1 tablespoon garlic powder
- ✓ 1 teaspoon of Himalayan salt
- ✓ 1 tablespoon barbecue seasoning

Directions:

Wash the kale and pick out leaves and snip with scissors to shape on rounds.

In a mixing bowl add all the ingredients and the shaped chips. Toss like a salad coating the chips with the ingredients.

Preheat oven to 300 degrees.

On a cookie sheet place chips and cook for 15

minutes, turning the chips once during the process.

Remember you can season these chips by using almost any combination of spices so experiment and see what you can concoct.

You can also just use larger leaves for a bigger chip.

7. KETO BROWNIES WITH NUTS

If you like brownies but can't have the sugar, try these. Unlike typical brownies they are healthy, yet still have a consistency and taste of decadent chocolate.

Ingredients:

- ✓ 1 avocado peeled and cubed
- ✓ ½ cup of coconut oil
- ✓ 2 tablespoons of coconut oil (grease the pan)
- ✓ ½ cup cocoa
- ✓ 2 tablespoons natural butter
- ✓ ½ cup coconut flour
- ✓ ½ teaspoon baking powder
- ✓ 1 teaspoon Stevia
- ✓ ½ cup dark baking chocolate
- ✓ 2 eggs, whisked with a dash of salt
- ✓ ½ teaspoon vanilla extract
- ✓ ½ cup almond slivers or walnuts

Directions:

In a medium mixing bowl, add the avocado and mash first. Now add the rest of the ingredients and beat with a hand mixer on medium for about 2 minutes. Preheat oven to 350 degrees.

In a brownie pan, add coconut oil to grease the pan. Next pour the brownie mix and use a spatula to smooth it into the pan. Bake for 15 minutes and let cool for 1 hour before eating.

 If you want to add a topping, use 1 cup heavy whipping cream, 1 teaspoon vanilla and 1 teaspoon Stevia to a cold bowl.

Mix on high until whipped cream consistency. Add to brownies.

8. CUCUMBER BOATS WITH CREAM CHEESE & RASPBERRIES

This simple recipe will actually surprise you because it tastes decadent but is really a tasty snack that is filling:

Ingredients:

- ✓ 2 medium cucumbers, cut in half and carefully peeled

- ✓ 1 package of Philly cream cheese

- ✓ 1 pinch of salt per cucumber

- ✓ ½ cup whipping cream

- ✓ 1 dash of Stevia

The Raspberry filling:

- ✓ ½ cup raspberries, strained through a collander, no seeds

- ✓ ¼ cup water, warm

- ✓ 1 teaspoon Stevia

- ✓ 1 pinch of cinnamon

- ✓ 1 teaspoon of Jello mix, red

Directions:

Using a spoon dig out a "trench" so that the cucumber boat will be formed and maximize what it can hold. Add the remnants of the cucumber to a mixing bowl and combine all of the first ingredients.

In a second mixing bowl combine all the raspberry topping mix. Blend and then add to the first set of ingredients and mix by hand again.

Now spoon the filling into the cucumber boats and serve.

9. QUICK VANILLA WHITE CHOCOLATE CUPCAKES

These are essentially mix, pour and bake and eat. Can't get much simpler and you will still be 100% on track for your new Keto Lifestyle.

Ingredients:

- ✓ ½ cup unsweetened white chocolate
- ✓ ½ cup coconut flour
- ✓ ¼ cup coconut oil
- ✓ 2 tablespoons coconut oil for cupcake wells
- ✓ 1 teaspoon Stevia
- ✓ 3 tablespoons coconut flour
- ✓ 1 teaspoon vanilla extract
- ✓ ½ teaspoon baking powder
- ✓ 1 scoop good quality vanilla protein powder
- ✓ 1 egg

Directions:

In a mixing bowl combine all the ingredients and beat with a hand mixer on high for 1 minute.

Preheat oven to 350 degrees.

In a cupcake tray, grease each well with coconut oil and pour the batter about half way into each well.

Cook for 15 minutes and let stand for 30 minutes to cool.

You can add almond slivers for additional taste and garnish.

CONCLUSION

Wow! What an amazing cooking journey we have had together!

As you can see, we have covered lots of great recipes that are not only tasty, but filled with nutrition and flavor.

It was my goal to also give you a set of core ingredients so that as you cooked, you began to see how many of these ingredients are used again and again.

This helps you not only learn how to cook, but to simplify your life and raise your skills, -- as well as make your shopping list much easier when it comes time to get what you need for cooking.

Remember that you need to keep the fat content up in these recipes so follow the directions carefully.

If a recipe does not call for many additional fats, this is because it can be found in the food itself, like the brownie recipe with avocados as a main ingredient.

I hope you learned a lot about Keto cooking here. I promise you if you follow these recipes you will love the foods and grow healthier as long as you always purchase the best organic components for each recipe.

You should also experiment with your own recipes using core cooking principles you have learned in this cookbook.

You will find that over time, you will become quite skilled with cooking these dishes and you will hardly need to consult the recipes because this book was laid out that way for overlapping cooking knowledge.

Best Regards,
David F. Wilson

www.ingramcontent.com/pod-product-compliance
Lightning Source LLC
Chambersburg PA
CBHW051437250726
48655CB00001B/100